2009
DIABETES ESSENTIALS

Fourth Edition

James H. O'Keefe, Jr., MD, FACC
Director, Preventive Cardiology
Mid-America Heart Institute
Professor of Medicine
University of Missouri School of Medicine
Kansas City, Missouri

David S. H. Bell, MB, FACE
Former Clinical Professor of Medicine
University of Alabama at Birmingham School of Medicine
Birmingham, Alabama

Kathleen L. Wyne, MD, PhD, FACE
Director of Clinical Research, Diabetes Research Center
The Methodist Hospital Research Institute
Weill Medical College, Cornell University
The Methodist Hospital
Houston, Texas

JONES AND BARTLETT PUBLISHERS
Sudbury, Massachusetts
BOSTON   TORONTO   LONDON   SINGAPORE

World Headquarters

Jones and Bartlett Publishers
40 Tall Pine Drive
Sudbury, MA 01776
978-443-5000
info@jbpub.com
www.jbpub.com

Jones and Bartlett Publishers
Canada
6339 Ormindale Way
Mississauga, ON L5V 1J2
CANADA

Jones and Bartlett Publishers
International
Barb House, Barb Mews
London W6 7PA
UK

Jones and Bartlett's books and products are available through most bookstores and online booksellers. To contact Jones and Bartlett Publishers directly, call 800-832-0034, fax 978-443-8000, or visit our website at www.jbpub.com.

Substantial discounts on bulk quantities of Jones and Bartlett's publications are available to corporations, professional associations, and other qualified organizations. For details and specific discount information, contact the special sales department at Jones and Bartlett via the above contact information or send an email to special-sales@jbpub.com.

The authors, editor, and publisher have made every effort to provide accurate information. However, they are not responsible for errors, omissions, or for any outcomes related to the use of the contents of this book and take no responsibility for the use of the products and procedures described. Treatments and side effects described in this book may not be applicable to all people; likewise, some people may require a dose or experience a side effect that is not described herein. Drugs and medical devices are discussed that may have limited availability controlled by the Food and Drug Administration (FDA) for use only in a research study or clinical trial. Research, clinical practice, and government regulations often change the accepted standard in this field. When consideration is being given to use of any drug in the clinical setting, the health care provider or reader is responsible for determining FDA status of the drug, reading the package insert, and reviewing prescribing information for the most up-to-date recommendations on dose, precautions, and contraindications, and determining the appropriate usage for the product. This is especially important in the case of drugs that are new or seldom used.

6048

ISBN: 978-0-7637-6608-5

Printed in the United States of America
13 12 11 10 09   10 9 8 7 6 5 4 3 2 1

ABOUT THE AUTHORS

 James H. O'Keefe, Jr., M.D., is the Director of Preventive Cardiology at the Mid America Heart Institute and Professor of Medicine at the University of Missouri in Kansas City. His postgraduate training included a cardiology fellowship at Mayo Clinic in Rochester, Minnesota. He has written 150 articles and 6 books on cardiovascular medicine, and he lectures extensively on the role of therapeutic lifestyle changes and drug therapy in cardiovascular risk reduction. He is actively involved in patient care.

 David S. H. Bell, MB, is a former Clinical Professor of Medicine at the University of Alabama at Birmingham, School of Medicine, and is a leading authority on the prevention and treatment of type 2 diabetes. During his distinguished career, he has contributed more than 260 articles to the medical literature. He is an active researcher and has served as Director of the Endocrine Clinical Research Program at the University of Alabama Birmingham. Dr. Bell speaks nationally and internationally on the treatment of type 2 diabetes and its complications, and he is currently or has been a member of the editorial boards of Endocrine Practice, Treatments in Endocrinology, Diabetes, Obesity and Metabolism, and Endocrine Today. He is a recipient of the Distinguished Clinician Award from the American College of Endocrinology for outstanding contribution as a master educator and clinician and the Seale Harris Award from the Southern Medical Association for superior contributions to the art and science of diabetes and endocrinology.

 Kathleen L. Wyne, MD, PhD, is the Director of Clinical Research for the Diabetes Research Institute of Weill Medical College, Cornell University, in Houston, Texas. Dr. Wyne is actively involved in basic science and clinical research. Her main research interests include studying the relationship between inflammation and insulin resistance and prevention of diabetes, especially in minority populations. In 1999 she received a Career Development Award from the Juvenile Diabetes Research Foundation International, and in 2000 she received a research grant from the same organization. Dr. Wyne has contributed many articles to the medical literature and lectures extensively on lipid metabolism and diabetes treatment. She is actively involved in patient care.

TABLES AND FIGURES

TABLE OF CONTENTS

CONTRIBUTORS

David S. H. Bell, MB
Clinical Professor of Medicine
University of Alabama Birmingham
Birmingham, Alabama

George L. Bakris, MD†
Professor of Preventive Medicine
Director, Hypertension/Clinical
  Research Center
Rush University Medical Center
Chicago, Illinois

Christie M. Ballantyne, MD*
Clinical Director, Section of Atherosclerosis
Professor of Medicine
Baylor College of Medicine
Houston, Texas

Mark S. Freed, MD
Cardiologist
President and Editor-in-Chief
Physicians' Press
Royal Oak, Michigan

Janet Haskin, PharmD
Clinical Coordinator
Del Sol Medical Center
El Paso, Texas
Diabetes Drug Summaries

Antonio M. Gotto, Jr, MD, DPhil*
The Stephen and Suzanne Weiss Dean
Professor of Medicine
Provost for Medical Affairs
The Weill Medical College of Cornell University
New York, New York

James H. O'Keefe, Jr, MD
Director, Preventive Cardiology
Mid America Heart Institute
Clinical Professor of Medicine
University of Missouri School of Medicine
Kansas City, Missouri

David M. Safley, MD
Cardiologist
Mid America Heart Institute
Kansas City, Missouri
Clinical Trials

Kathleen L. Wyne, MD, PhD
Assistant Professor
Division of Endocrinology and Metabolism
University of Texas Southwestern Medical
Center
Dallas, Texas

---

* Portions of Chapter 7, "Control of Dyslipidemia in Type 2 Diabetes," and Chapter 9, "Other Measures to Reduce Atherothrombosis," adapted from *Dyslipidemia Essentials*, by Ballantyne CM, O'Keefe JH, Jr, Gotto AM, Jr, Physicians' Press, 2008, Royal Oak, Michigan

† Portions of Chapter 8, "Control of Hypertension in Type 2 Diabetes," adapted from *Handbook of Diabetic Hypertension*, by Bell DSH, O'Keefe JH, Jr, Bakris GL, Physicians' Press, 2006, Royal Oak, Michigan

ACKNOWLEDGMENTS

To accomplish the task of presenting the data compiled in this reference, a small, dedicated team of professionals was assembled. We wish to acknowledge Monica Crowder Kaufman for her important contribution, Norman Lyle for cover design, and Mark S. Freed, MD, President and Editor-in-Chief of Physicians' Press, for his vision, commitment, and guidance.

James H. O'Keefe, Jr, MD
Kathleen L. Wyne, MD, PhD
David S.H. Bell, MB

NOTICE

ABBREVIATIONS

AACE/ACE	American Association of Clinical Endocrinologists/American College of Endocrinology	gm	gram
		GFR	glomerular filtration rate
ACE	angiotensin converting enzyme	GP	glycoprotein
ACS	acute coronary syndrome	HbA_{1c}	hemoglobin A_{1c}
ADA	American Diabetes Association	HDL	high-density lipoprotein
ADP	adenosine diphosphate	Hgb	hemoglobin
AHA	American Heart Association	IFG	impaired fasting glucose
ARB	angiotensin receptor blocker	IGT	impaired glucose tolerance
ATP	Adult Treatment Panel (National Cholesterol Education Program)	IV	intravenous
		kg	kilogram
		L	liter
BID	twice daily	LDL	low-density lipoprotein
BMI	body mass index	LFT	liver function test
BP	blood pressure	Lp(a)	lipoprotein(a)
BUN	blood urea nitrogen	LV	left ventricular; left ventricle
CABG	coronary artery bypass grafting	LVH	left ventricular hypertrophy
CHD	coronary heart disease	max	maximum
CI	contraindication	mcg	microgram
CK	creatine kinase	mcL	microliter
CNS	central nervous system	mg	milligram
COPD	chronic obstructive pulmonary disease	MI	myocardial infarction
		min	minute
CrCl	creatinine clearance	mL	milliliter
CRP	C-reactive protein	NCEP	National Cholesterol Education Program
DHA	docosahexaenoic acid		
DKA	diabetic ketoacidosis	NRT	nicotine replacement therapy
dL	deciliter	NYHA	New York Heart Association
DPP-4	dipeptidyl peptidase-4	OGTT	oral glucose tolerance test
DVT	deep venous thrombosis	PAI-1	plasminogen activator inhibitor-1
EASD	European Association for the Study of Diabetes	PCI	percutaneous coronary intervention
ECG	electrocardiogram	PE	pulmonary embolism
e.g.	for example	PO	per os - by mouth; oral
EPA	eicosapentaenoic acid	PPAR	peroxisome proliferator-activated receptor
FBG	fasting blood glucose		
FDA	Food and Drug Administration	q__h	every __ hours
FPG	fasting plasma glucose	q__d	every __ days
GDM	gestational diabetes mellitus	TG	triglyceride
GI	gastrointestinal	TIA	transient ischemic attack
GIP	glucose-dependent insulinotropic polypeptide	TLC	therapeutic lifestyle changes
		TID	three times daily
		TZD	thiazolidinedione
GLP-1	glucagon-like peptide-1	US	United States

Chapter 1

Diabetes Essentials

Diabetes mellitus is a global public health problem of epidemic proportions, and its incidence is on the rise. In the United States (US) alone, approximately 21 million adults have diabetes and 35% of adults have prediabetes or diabetes (Diabetes Care 2006;29:1263-1268). Worldwide, more than 150 million adults have diabetes, a number the World Health Organization expects to double over the next 20 years.

Diabetes is associated with accelerated atherosclerosis and a prothrombotic state, markedly increasing the risk of myocardial infarction (MI), stroke, peripheral arterial disease, and heart failure. Seventy-five percent of individuals with diabetes die from cardiovascular disease, and diabetic subjects without known coronary artery disease have the same cardiovascular prognosis as nondiabetic subjects with coronary artery disease. Of patients admitted to hospitals in the US, 43% have diabetes. Diabetes is also the leading cause of adult blindness, end-stage renal disease, and nontraumatic leg amputation. Diabetes confers an equivalent cardiovascular risk to aging 15 years (Lancet 2006;368:29-36). Compared to death rates for cardiovascular disease, stroke, and cancer, which have remained stable or have declined since 1980, death rates for diabetes have increased by 30% during the same time period. The annual cost of diabetes in terms of medical care and lost productivity exceeds $130 billion in the United States alone.

Measures aimed at slowing the progression of atherosclerosis, stabilizing rupture-prone plaques, and preventing arterial thrombosis can reduce the risk of cardiac death, MI, stroke, revascularization procedures, and peripheral arterial disease by 50%-80%. The lower the hemoglobin A_{1c}, even within the normal range, the lower the risk of a cardiovascular event and cardiac and all-cause mortality. Despite these benefits, only 7.3% of individuals with diabetes meet national guidelines for control of hemoglobin A_{1c}, cholesterol and blood pressure, and tens of thousands of lives are lost each year from failure to implement established measures. The American Diabetes Association (ADA) has estimated that, in the US alone, if 80% of individuals with type 2 diabetes achieved five recommended ADA treatment goals over

Table 1.1. ADA Treatment Goals for Individuals with Type 2 Diabetes

- Hemoglobin A1c < 7%
- Blood pressure < 130/80 mmHg
- LDL cholesterol < 100 mg/dL
- HDL > 40 mg/dL for men and > 50 mg/dL for women
- Use of aspirin, 81 mg daily

the next 30 years (Table 1.1), there would be 5 million fewer heart attacks, 1.2 million fewer cases of kidney failure, 1.8 million fewer cases of blindness, and 1.8 million fewer premature deaths. In addition, more than $150 billion in medical costs could be saved. *Diabetes Essentials* incorporates the latest guidelines and trials into a practical, concise, authoritative guide to the diagnosis, evaluation, prevention, and management of type 2 diabetes, the most prevalent form of the disease.

Overview of Diabetes Mellitus

A. Description. Diabetes mellitus is the most common endocrine disorder in men and women. It is caused by an absolute lack of insulin (type 1) or a relative lack of insulin (type 2) that is insufficient to overcome insulin resistance. Manifestations include hyperglycemia, other metabolic derangements, and long-term damage to blood vessels, eyes, nerves, kidneys, and the heart (Table 1.2). Diabetes is a leading cause of cardiac death, nonfatal MI, heart failure, and stroke; it is also the most common cause of adult blindness, end-stage renal disease, nontraumatic leg amputation, and neuropathy in the United States.

B. Prevalence. Approximately 21 million Americans and 150 million individuals worldwide have diabetes, a number projected to double by the year 2025. Over a 10-year period from 1990-2000, the prevalence of diabetes increased by 49%, from 4.9% to 7.3% in the US. The US Centers for Disease Control and Prevention estimates that in the United States, 8.6% of adults have diabetes and 800,000 new cases of diabetes will be diagnosed in the upcoming year. Data from the National Health Interview Survey estimate that the lifetime risk of developing diabetes for

Table 1.2. Complications of Type 2 Diabetes

Acute Complications
    Diabetic ketoacidosis
    Hyperosmolar coma
    Hypoglycemia

Long-Term Complications
Microvascular
    Retinopathy
    Nephropathy
    Peripheral/autonomic neuropathy
Macrovascular
    Coronary heart disease
    Cerebrovascular disease
    Peripheral arterial disease
Other
    Decreased resistance to infection (with hyperglycemia)
    Skin changes
    Poor wound healing
    Cataracts
    Glaucoma
    Infertility
    Non-alcoholic steatosis/steatohepatitis (complication of insulin resistance)

individuals born in the U.S. in 2000 is 33% for men and 39% for females, resulting in large reductions in life expectancy and quality of life (JAMA 2003;290:1884-89). Stated another way, babies born in the US today have a one in three lifetime risk of developing diabetes and, if born into a high-risk ethnic group, the risk exceeds one in two. In addition, more than 5.5 million cases of diabetes in the U.S. are undiagnosed, and 26% of the American population (44% of those over age 60) have either impaired fasting glucose (prediabetes) or insulin resistance (metabolic syndrome), substantially increasing the risk of diabetes and cardiovascular events (Chapter 2). Elderly persons and certain ethnic groups (African Americans, Asians, Hispanics, Native Americans, Pacific Islanders) are at higher risk for developing diabetes. Today, 11% of American teenagers are prediabetic, and 10% of diabetes diagnosed in individuals under age 18 is type 2. In high-risk ethnic groups, as much as 50% of diabetes developing under age 18 is type 2 diabetes.

Notwithstanding, the prevalence of insulin resistance, beta cell dysfunction, and overt type 2 diabetes all increase with age. In addition to an aging population, the growing epidemic of diabetes has been attributed to increasing rates of obesity, declining levels of physical activity, and a high-carbohydrate, calorie dense diet consisting mostly of processed synthetic foods.

C. Classification of Diabetes (Table 1.3)

1. **Type 1 Diabetes.** This form of diabetes accounts for 5-10% of all cases. The vast majority of type 1 diabetes is caused by cell-mediated autoimmune destruction of the pancreatic islet beta-cells, resulting in failure of the pancreas to produce insulin and an absolute insulin deficiency. A family history of diabetes is less common than with type 2 diabetes. Twin studies show that 30-50% of the initially non-affected monozygotic twins will develop type 1 diabetes. Autoantibodies to islet cells, glutamic acid decarboxylase (GAD) and insulin are often present, and the risk for other autoimmune diseases is increased (Graves disease, Hashimoto's thyroiditis, Addison's disease, pernicious anemia). A small minority of cases are idiopathic (not autoimmune) in origin. Type 1 diabetes usually presents with the acute onset of symptoms (polyuria, polydipsia, polyphagia, weight loss) and disproportionately affects young people (70% of cases occur by age 20, though it can occur at any age), the majority of whom are not obese. Life-long insulin therapy is required for survival. Persons with type 1 diabetes are prone to diabetic ketoacidosis (DKA) because of an absolute deficiency of endogenous insulin, and DKA may be the initial manifestation of their disease. The terms "insulin dependent diabetes mellitus (IDDM)," "type I diabetes" (using the Roman numeral), and "juvenile onset diabetes mellitus" are no longer used to describe this condition.

2. **Type 2 Diabetes.** This form of diabetes accounts for 90-95% of all cases. Type 2 diabetes is caused by insulin resistance combined with an inability of the pancreatic beta cells to produce sufficient insulin to overcome the insulin resistance. Affected individuals almost always have a family history, particularly on the maternal side, possibly due to a defect in the cofactor for the PPAR-gamma receptor

Table 1.3. Etiologic Classification of Diabetes Mellitus

Type 1 diabetes[†][*]
- Immune-mediated (vast majority)
- Idiopathic

Type 2 diabetes[‡][*]

Other specific types
- Genetic defects of beta-cell function or insulin action
- Diseases of the exocrine pancreas (pancreatitis, trauma/pancreatectomy, neoplasia, cystic fibrosis, hemochromatosis, fibrocalculous pancreatopathy)
- Endocrinopathies (acromegaly, Cushing's syndrome, glucagonoma, pheochromocytoma, hyperthyroidism, somatostatinoma, aldosteronoma, others)
- Drug- or chemical-induced (pentamidine, nicotinic acid, glucocorticoids, thyroid hormone, diazoxide, beta-adrenergic agonists, thiazides, dilantin, alpha-interferon, others)
- Infections (congenital rubella, cytomegalovirus, Coxsackie B, others)
- Uncommon forms of immune-mediated diabetes ("Stiff-man" syndrome, anti-insulin receptor antibodies, others)
- Other genetic syndromes sometimes associated with diabetes (Down's syndrome, Klinefelter's syndrome, Turner's syndrome, Wolfram's syndrome, Friedreich's ataxia, Huntington's chorea, Laurence-Moon-Biedl syndrome, myotonic dystrophy, porphyria, Prader-Willi syndrome, others)

Gestational diabetes mellitus (GDM)

† Beta cell destruction usually resulting in absolute insulin deficiency
‡ May range from predominantly insulin resistance with relative insulin deficiency to a predominantly secretory defect with insulin resistance
* Patients with any form of diabetes may require insulin treatment at some stage of their disease. Use of insulin does not, by itself, classify the patient.

From: The Expert Committee on the Diagnosis and Classification of Diabetes Mellitus, from the American Diabetes Association. Diabetes Care 2007;30(suppl 1):S4-S41.

in the mitochondria; this genetic predisposition in conjunction with behavioral and environmental risk factors— advanced age, obesity, and sedentary lifestyle—are responsible for the development of insulin resistance and diabetes. If one monozygotic twin develops type 2 diabetes, then over 90% of the initially non-affected twins will also develop the disease. In contrast to type 1 diabetes, type 2 diabetes historically affects people over the age of 40 (but is now seen as young as 3 years old), many of whom are obese, and autoimmune destruction of pancreatic islet beta cells does not occur. Less than one-third of type 2 diabetic patients will ultimately require insulin therapy, although the likelihood increases in proportion to the duration of diabetes. To achieve/maintain glycemic goal, many patients with type 2 diabetes will need insulin therapy within 10 years. Episodes of spontaneous DKA are rare, but may develop during extreme stress or severe illness (Table 1.4), particularly in African Americans and Latinos. Importantly, early symptoms (fatigue, postprandial hypoglycemia) are often overlooked or ignored, and type 2 diabetes can go undetected for years, only to first present with a microvascular or macrovascular complication (e.g., MI, stroke, loss of vision, peripheral neuropathy). Diet, exercise, and weight loss can improve insulin resistance and occasionally appear to reverse type 2 diabetes, particularly in some obese people. Following bariatric surgery, increased GLP-1 production stimulates growth and suppresses apoptosis (programmed cell death) of insulin-producing beta cells, resulting in rates of recovery from diabetes of up to 75%. The term "non-insulin dependent diabetes mellitus (NIDDM)" is no longer used to describe this condition.

3. **Gestational Diabetes.** Gestational diabetes is defined as glucose intolerance that is first identified during pregnancy. The definition applies regardless of whether insulin or only diet modification is used for treatment or whether the condition persists after pregnancy. It does not exclude the possibility that unrecognized glucose intolerance may have antedated or started concomitantly with the pregnancy or that type 1 diabetes may develop during pregnancy. In the U.S., approximately 7% of all pregnancies are complicated by gestational diabetes, usually during the second or third trimester of pregnancy when elevated levels of human placental lactogen (HPL) raise insulin resistance. Hyperglycemia may be mild and asymptomatic, but treatment with insulin is often required to prevent fetal morbidity and mortality. Metformin and glyburide have been used off-label for gestational diabetes. Glucose tolerance typically reverts toward normal early in the postpartum period, but 35% of women are subsequently diagnosed with type 2 diabetes within 5-10 years. Pregnancy provides a "stress test" for the pancreas with suboptimal insulin secretion and warns that unless preventive

measures (especially weight loss) are initiated the risk of type 2 diabetes in later life will be greatly increased.

4. **Other Types of Diabetes.** This category includes diabetes caused by genetic defects in beta-cell function or insulin action, genetic mitochondrial defects (maternal inherited diabetes mellitus plus deafness), diseases of the exocrine pancreas (e.g., hemochromatosis),

Table 1.4. Clinical Features of Diabetes Mellitus

	Type 1 Diabetes	**Type 2 Diabetes**
Prevalence (US)	0.4%	8.6%
Primary defect	Autoimmune (common) or idiopathic (rare) destruction of pancreatic islet beta-cells; insulin deficiency is usually absolute	Genetic, environmental factors resulting in insulin resistance with a combined insulin secretory defect; insulin deficiency is relative
Presentation	Acute onset of symptoms (polyuria, polydipsia, polyphagia, weight loss); often acutely ill; may present with ketoacidosis. Diagnosis is made soon after symptoms develop. Age at presentation < 20 years in 70% of cases; most are not obese	Subtle symptoms may go unnoticed/undetected for years. Vascular complication or neuropathy can be presenting complaint. Age at presentation is typically > 45 years; most are obese. Ketoacidosis is rare but may occur during severe illness/stress
Treatment	Insulin is required for survival. Hypoglycemia occurs more often in type 1 diabetes	Diet, exercise, and weight loss are sufficient in some and may reverse the condition. Most require oral drug therapy; many require > 1 agent. Insulin is eventually required in many

endocrinopathies (e.g., Cushing's syndrome, hyperthyroidism), drug/chemical-induced diabetes, and other conditions (Table 1.3).

5. **Other Disorders of Glucose Regulation.** Impaired glucose tolerance (IGT) and impaired fasting glucose (IFG) are risk factors for diabetes. These conditions are also referred to as "prediabetes," as at least 25% of affected individuals eventually develop type 2 diabetes. All persons with IGT or IFG should receive instruction on therapeutic lifestyle changes (Chapter 4). A fasting plasma glucose is recommended annually to detect the onset of diabetes and the need for more aggressive therapy. Several interventions have been shown to reduce the progression from prediabetes to diabetes, including diet/exercise (58% reduction), rosiglitazone (60% reduction), metformin (31% reduction), acarbose (25% reduction), and bariatric surgery (70% reduction) (Chapter 2). Studies are in progress (e.g., NAVIGATOR [ARB and nateglinide], ACT NOW [pioglitazone]) to determine whether other pharmacological interventions can prevent or delay the development of type 2 diabetes.

D. **Presentation.** The most common presentation of type 1 diabetes is polyuria with polydipsia. Other symptoms include weight loss despite increased appetite, blurred vision, drowsiness, poor stamina, nausea, frequent skin and bladder infections, and Candida vaginitis in women. In type 1 diabetes, symptoms usually develop abruptly over weeks, and patients may be acutely ill on presentation. In type 2 diabetes, symptoms may gradually appear over months to years, making this condition easy to overlook or ignore, and patients often do not recognize that they are unwell until a dramatic improvement in "well being" occurs with diabetic therapy. Reactive hypoglycemia — due to a loss of first-phase insulin response, post-prandial hyperglycemia, and hyperinsulinemia leading to late hypoglycemia — is often present early in the course of type 2 diabetes. Chronic and undiagnosed hyperglycemia in type 2 diabetes can induce pathological changes in organ tissues before symptoms are recognized. By the time diabetes is diagnosed, a microvascular or neurologic complication is already present in 40% of patients. Occasionally, the initial manifestation of diabetes is a microvascular complication (retinopathy, nephropathy, neuropathy), a macrovascular complication (MI, stroke, CHF, peripheral vascular disease), or a medical emergency that can threaten survival without hospitalization and treatment (DKA, nonketotic hyperosmolar coma). Approximately two-thirds of subjects presenting with stable CHD or acute coronary syndrome have either type 2 diabetes or impaired glucose tolerance (Am J Cardiol 2005;96:363-5). In patients who do not have diabetes at the time of their first MI, over the next 5 years the risk of developing type 2 diabetes is increased 2-3–fold in men and 3-4–fold in women (Diabet Med 2005;22:1334-7).

E. Screening for Diabetes. Many type 2 diabetic subjects are asymptomatic and can go undiagnosed for years, during which time pathological changes can develop in non-insulin sensitive tissues due to chronic exposure to hyperglycemia. Early diagnosis and treatment of type 2 diabetes can prevent the development of microvascular and macrovascular complications. Therefore, the American Diabetes Association recommends screening all high-risk individuals for diabetes (Table 1.5).

F. Diagnosis (Table 1.6). The American Diabetes Association requires the presence of one of the following criteria for the diagnosis of diabetes (Diabetes Care 2008;31[suppl 1]:S12-S55):
  - Unequivocal elevation of plasma glucose concentrations on more than one occasion associated with classic symptoms of diabetes
  - Elevation of fasting plasma glucose (FPG) on more than one occasion
  - Elevation of plasma glucose following a standardized oral glucose tolerance test

G. Management of Diabetes. Traditional therapeutic efforts aimed predominantly at normalizing elevated glucose levels without aggressively controlling other modifiable risk factors associated with insulin resistance have proven inadequate for reducing cardiovascular events in type 2 diabetes. Optimal management requires a coordinated team approach aimed at intensive glycemic control, improving insulin sensitivity, treatment of dyslipidemia and hypertension, management of diabetes-related complications, and patient education. Such an approach has sustained benefits on cardiovascular prognosis (N Engl J Med 2008;358:580-591).

Table 1.5. Screening for Pre-Diabetes and Diabetes in Asymptomatic Individuals*

Testing should be considered for age ≥ 45 years, particularly in those with a BMI ≥ 25 kg/m²†. If the test is normal, it should be repeated at 3-year intervals. Testing should be considered at a younger age or be carried out more frequently in overweight (BMI ≥ 25 kg/m²†) individuals with additional risk factors:

- first-degree relative with diabetes
- habitually physically inactive
- member of a high-risk ethnic population (e.g., African American, Hispanic American, Native American, Asian American, Pacific Islander)
- delivery of a baby weighing > 9 lbs or history of gestational diabetes
- hypertension (BP ≥ 140/90 mmHg)
- HDL cholesterol ≤ 35 mg/dL or triglyceride ≥ 250 mg/dL
- polycystic ovary syndrome
- impaired glucose tolerance or impaired fasting glucose on previous testing
- history of cardiovascular disease

* Fasting plasma glucose or an oral glucose tolerance test may be used to diagnose diabetes (Table 1.6)

† May not be correct for all ethnic groups

From: Standards of Medical Care in Diabetes. The American Diabetes Association. Diabetes Care 2008;31(suppl 1):S12-S55.

H. **Natural History and Prognosis.** Type 2 diabetes is a chronic, progressive disorder resulting in gradual loss of pancreatic islet beta cell function and the need for escalating drug therapy over time. If left unchecked, rising HbA$_{1c}$ levels increase the risk of microvascular and macrovascular complications. The lifetime risk of developing diabetes for individuals born in the U.S. today is one in three, and the presence of diabetes markedly reduces both long-term survival and quality of life. For diabetes diagnosed at age 40, long-term survival and quality of survival are reduced by approximately 12.5 years and 20 years, respectively (JAMA 2003;290:1884-1889). Preventive strategies can delay the onset/slow the progression of diabetes-related complications (Chapters 2, 6-9).

Table 1.6. Criteria for the Diagnosis of Diabetes Mellitus

Category	Fasting Plasma Glucose (mg/dL)	2-Hour Plasma Glucose[†] (mg/dL)	Casual Plasma Glucose[††] (mg/dL)
Normoglycemia	< 100	< 140	–
IFG/IGT	100-125 / –	– / 140-199	–
Diabetes	≥ 126*	≥ 200	> 200 with symptoms of diabetes*

IFG = impaired fasting glucose, IGT = impaired glucose tolerance

* A diagnosis of diabetes must be confirmed on a subsequent day. The fasting plasma glucose test is preferred because of ease of administration, convenience, acceptability to patients, and lower cost. Fasting is defined as no caloric intake for at least 8 hours.

† This test requires the use of a glucose load containing the equivalent of 75 gm anhydrous glucose in water followed by plasma glucose measurement 2 hours later

†† Anytime of day without regard to last meal

From: The American Diabetes Association. Diabetes Care 2008;31(suppl 1):S12-S55.

Chapter 2

Metabolic Syndrome, Insulin Resistance, Prediabetes, and Prevention of Type 2 Diabetes

A. **The Metabolic Syndrome.** The metabolic syndrome is characterized by a cluster of metabolic abnormalities that increases cardiovascular risk, chief among them being insulin resistance. Approximately 24% (47 million) of adult Americans have the metabolic syndrome, and the prevalence of this disorder is escalating. The diagnosis requires the presence of at least 3 of 5 major criteria, as defined by the National Cholesterol Education Program Adult Treatment Panel III (Table 2.1). However, since waist circumference is often measured inaccurately or not measure at all in clinical practice, the frequency of the metabolic syndrome may be underestimated. A practical guide to the presence of the metabolic syndrome is a triglyceride-to-HDL ratio > 3.5. Individuals with the metabolic syndrome are at increased risk of developing diabetes and cardiovascular events, the latter due to accelerated atherosclerosis, inflammation, hypercoagulability, and endothelial dysfunction (Table 2.2). Compared to men without any of the 5 features of the metabolic syndrome, those with 4 or 5 features have a 25-fold increased risk of new diabetes and a 4-fold increased risk of coronary heart disease; the presence of inflammation, manifest as elevated C-reactive protein, further

Table 2.1. Criteria for the Diagnosis of the Metabolic Syndrome*

- Abdominal obesity: waist circumference > 102 cm (40 in) in men or > 88 cm (35 in) in women
- Triglycerides ≥ 150 mg/dL
- HDL cholesterol < 40 mg/dL in men or < 50 mg/dL in women
- Blood pressure ≥ 130/85 mmHg
- Impaired fasting glucose (fasting glucose 100-125 mg/dL)

* Clinical identification of the metabolic syndrome requires the presence of at least 3 of 5 factors. The metabolic syndrome is associated with an increased risk of new diabetes and cardiovascular events. From: Circulation 2004;109:433-438.

Table 1. Oral Glycemic Agents Used for Type 2 Diabetes

Drug Class	Antidiabetic Agents	Mechanism of Action
Biguanides	Metformin (Glucophage)	Decreased hepatic glucose output
Thiazolidinediones (TZDs)	Rosiglitazone (Avandia) Pioglitazone (Actos)	Increased insulin sensitivity; preservation of beta cell function
Alpha-glucosidase inhibitors	Acarbose (Precose) Miglitol (Glyset)	Delayed GI absorption of carbohydrates
Insulin secretagogues *Sulfonylureas*	Chlorpropamide (Diabinese) Glipizide (Glucotrol/XL) Glyburide (DiaBeta, Micronase, Glynase) Glimepiride (Amaryl)	Increased insulin release
Glitinides	Nateglinide (Starlix) Repaglinide (Prandin)	Increased insulin release
Dipeptidyl peptidase-4 (DPP-4) inhibitor	Sitagliptin (Januvia)	Increased GLP-1 levels; augmentation of glucose-stimulated insulin release and suppression of glucagon production; preservation of beta cell function
Combination TZD + biguanide	Rosiglitazone + metformin (Avandamet) Pioglitazone + metformin (Actoplusmet)	Increased insulin sensitivity; decreased hepatic glucose output; preservation of beta cell function
Combination sulfonylurea + biguanide	Glipizide + metformin (Metaglip) Glyburide + metformin (Glucovance)	Increased insulin secretion; decreased hepatic glucose output
Combination TZD + sulfonylurea	Rosiglitazone + glimepiride (Avandaryl) Pioglitazone + glimepiride (Duetact)	Increased insulin secretion; increased insulin sensitivity; preservation of beta cell function
Combination DPP-4 inhibitor + metformin	Sitagliptin + metformin (Janumet)	See DPP-4 inhibitor, above; decreased hepatic glucose output

Glycemic Control in Type 2 Diabetes

James H. O'Keefe, Jr., MD, David S. H. Bell, MD
Kathleen L. Wyne, MD, PhD

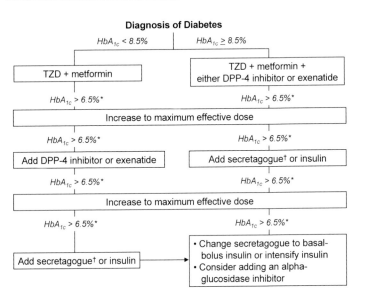

Figure 1. Initial Combination Therapy for Type 2 Diabetes

The authors favor an aggressive initial approach using a combination of drugs aimed at more than one mechanism to optimize glycemic control without causing severe or frequent hypoglycemic episodes. Reinforce lifestyle intervention at every visit

* Consider using a target $HbA_{1c} > 7.0\%$ (instead of 6.5%) for individuals with long-standing type 2 diabetes, significant coronary heart disease, and a predisposition to hypoglycemia. For initiation/titration of TZD, check HbA_{1c} at 6 months. For all other agents, check HbA_{1c} at 3 months

† Sulfonylurea or glitinide (nateglinide, repaglinide)

Table 2.2. Pathophysiological Changes Associated with the Metabolic Syndrome

Some degree of glucose intolerance
- Impaired fasting glucose: plasma glucose 100-125 mg/dL
- Impaired glucose intolerance: plasma glucose 140-199 mg/dL 2 hours after a 75-gram oral glucose challenge

Dyslipidemia
- Triglycerides > 150 mg/dL
- HDL cholesterol < 40 mg/dL (men), < 50 mg/dL (women)
- Increased small, dense, atherogenic LDL and ApoB particles
- Postprandial elevation of triglyceride-rich lipoproteins

Endothelial dysfunction
- Increased mononuclear cell adhesion
- Elevated plasma concentration of cellular adhesion molecules
- Impaired endothelial-dependent vasodilatation

Hemodynamic changes
- Augmented sympathetic nervous system activity
- Renal sodium retention
- Elevated blood pressure

Prothrombotic factors
- Increased plasminogen activator inhibitor-1
- Increased fibrinogen

Inflammation
- Increased C-reactive protein, white blood cells, cytokines, etc.

Increased plasma uric acid concentration

These changes increase the risk of cardiovascular disease

increases risk (Circulation 2003;108:414-419). Environmental factors, such as excessive intake of saturated fat, processed carbohydrate and calories; obesity; and sedentary lifestyle substantially increase the risk of developing the metabolic syndrome and type 2 diabetes. (Decades ago, diabetes was rare [< 1%] in the Inuit population, who followed a traditional hunter-gatherer lifestyle of extensive daily physical exertion. Today, after developing a more sedentary lifestyle and embracing a

Westernized diet of increased calories, processed carbohydrates, and trans fats, approximately 75% of Inuits are obese and 66% of Inuit women have type 2 diabetes.) Genetics also impact insulin sensitivity—offspring of individuals with type 2 diabetes, hypertension, or atherosclerosis have higher degrees of insulin resistance than offspring of healthy controls. With aging and obesity, mitochondrial function declines, worsening any genetic predisposition to insulin resistance.

The problem with the ATP III definition is lack of ethnic specific criteria for obesity. The International Diabetes Federation (IDF) recommended a new definition with a goal of emphasizing the role of central obesity and insulin resistance as causative factors. They suggested that the waist circumference plus any two additional factors, using the same metabolic criteria, be required to make the diagnosis of metabolic syndrome. Additionally, they created ethnic specific criteria for the measurement of waist circumference and recommended that ethnic group specific cut-points should be used for people of the same ethnic group regardless of where the person lives. This new definition helps to identify the metabolic syndrome in ethnic groups who are insulin resistant at lower BMIs than the general US population. In clinical practice, if the triglyceride-to-HDL ratio is greater than 3.5, then it is likely that the patient has insulin resistance and is at increased risk for cardiovascular disease and diabetes (Am J Cardiol 2005;96;399-404).

Treatment of the metabolic syndrome requires increased physical activity (Chapter 4), weight control (Chapter 4), and optimal management of hypertension and dyslipidemia (Chapters 7-8). The American College of Endocrinology has recommended that persons with the metabolic syndrome be treated to the same LDL target as those with diabetes (< 100 mg/dL). Diet modification, smoking cessation, and use of antiplatelet therapy and ACE inhibitors for high risk individuals are also indicated for overall cardiovascular health (Chapters 4, 9).

B. Insulin Resistance, Hyperinsulinemia, and Cardiovascular Disease. Insulin resistance is the underlying pathophysiological defect in both the metabolic syndrome and type 2 diabetes. Insulin resistance is characterized by marked impairment of insulin-stimulated glucose uptake by peripheral tissues. This is associated with a decrease in adiponectin production, and increases in adipocyte free fatty acid and cytokine production (TNFα, PAI-1, angiotensinogen, ilentin G [stimulates C-reactive protein production by liver], resistin, leptin), hepatic glucose production, insulin levels, and the risk of atherosclerotic vascular disease (Figure 2.1). Approximately 30% of the American population have insulin resistance, including 58% of persons with hypertension, 65% with coronary disease, and 85% with hypertriglyceridemia and low HDL cholesterol. Compared to persons with normal glucose homeostasis, insulin-resistant individuals with hyperinsulinemia or impaired fasting glucose are at increased risk of cardiovascular events (Figures 2.2, 2.3). The risk of non-alcoholic fatty liver disease, polycystic ovarian syndrome, and possibly several forms of cancer (e.g., breast, prostate) are increased as well. Insulin resistance is treated the same as the metabolic syndrome, with emphasis placed on improving insulin sensitivity through weight control and increased physical activity. Weight loss of as little as 5-10 pounds in overweight/obese individuals with insulin resistance can substantially improve insulin sensitivity, reduce plasma glucose levels, and improve manifestations of the metabolic syndrome. Substantial weight loss, as achieved with gastric bypass, results in normoglycemia for a sustained period in approximately 70%, though this may be due to improved beta cell function (see Chapter 5). Evolving evidence suggests that a low-glycemic load, high fiber diet with adequate amounts of monounsaturated and omega-3 fats and lean protein can improve satiety, dietary thermogenesis (basal metabolic rate), and insulin sensitivity. Non-fat dairy products, soy foods, and modest alcohol intake (not more than 1 drink per day in women or 2 drinks per day in men) can also improve insulin sensitivity (Table 2.3). Exercise lowers glucose levels acutely and for up to 48 hours after physical activity, lowers triglyceride levels, raises HDL levels, and facilitates weight loss. Among oral diabetic medications, thiazolidinediones (TZD's) directly improve insulin resistance. Other agents may indirectly improve insulin resistance by lowering glucose, and metformin improves insulin resistance by reducing food intake and body weight.

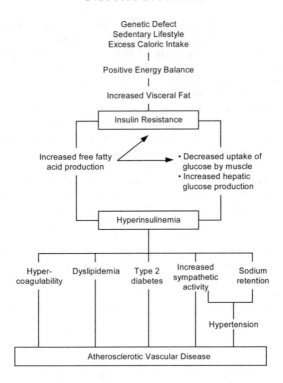

Figure 2.1. Insulin Resistance, Hyperinsulinemia, and Atherosclerosis

Sedentary lifestyle, poor diet, and obesity lead to insulin resistance, hyperinsulinemia, and increased risk of cardiovascular events.

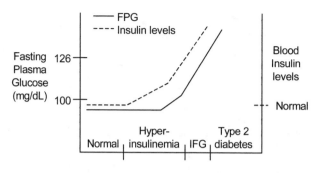

Figure 2.2. Insulin Levels and Glycemia in Type 2 Diabetes

As skeletal muscle becomes more resistant to insulin, increased insulin levels are required to maintain normal plasma glucose levels. Over time, elevated insulin levels are unable to keep pace with progressive insulin resistance, resulting in impaired fasting glucose (IFG). Insulin-resistant individuals often develop a cluster of cardiovascular risk factors (metabolic syndrome) that increases the risk of cardiac death, MI, and stroke (Table 2.2). Insulin levels may remain elevated early in type 2 diabetes but eventually decline due to loss of beta cell function (Figure 2.4). The "ticking clock" hypothesis states that atherosclerosis and increased risk of adverse events begin when insulin resistance develops, typically years to decades before type 2 diabetes is diagnosed.

C. **Importance of Postprandial Hyperglycemia on Cardiovascular Risk Factors, Atherosclerosis, and Cardiac Events.** Epidemiological data consistently demonstrate that postprandial hyperglycemia is an independent predictor of future cardiovascular events in diabetic and nondiabetic subjects (Figure 2.5). The cardiovascular toxicity of postprandial hyperglycemia appears to be mediated by oxidant stress, which is directly proportional to glucose and lipid excursions after a meal. This transient increase in free radical formation acutely triggers inflammation, endothelial dysfunction, hypercoagulability, sympathetic hyperactivity, and a cascade of other atherogenic changes (Figure 2.6).

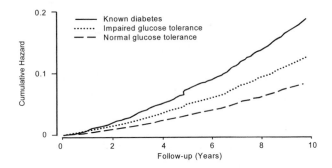

Figure 2.3. Insulin Resistance and Cardiovascular Risk

This risk of cardiovascular disease increases with the development of insulin resistance and hyperinsulinemia. Individuals with impaired glucose tolerance or the metabolic syndrome have cardiovascular risk that is intermediate between normal subjects and those with type 2 diabetes. From: Lancet 1999;354:617-621.

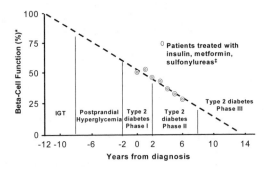

Figure 2.4. Loss of Pancreatic Beta Cell Function in UKPDS

IGT = impaired glucose tolerance. Typically, up to 50% of beta cell function has been lost by the time type 2 diabetes is diagnosed. After 15 years of diabetes, less than 10% of beta cells are functioning and insulin replacement therapy is often required.

* Dashed line shows extrapolation forward and backward from years 0-6 from diagnosis of diabetes based on Homeostasis Model Assessment data from UKPDS.

From: Diabetes Rev 1999;7:139-153.

Table 2.3. Effect of Dietary Modifications on Insulin Resistance

Improves Insulin Resistance	Worsens Insulin Resistance
Decreased caloric intake	High-glycemic load foods
Minimally-processed vegetables, fruits, legumes, and whole grains	Trans fats and saturated fats
Fiber	Excess calorie intake
Lean protein	Highly-processed, easily digested foods
Light-to-moderate alcohol intake	
Nuts	
Non-fat dairy	
Cinnamon	

Early studies found that blunting of postprandial spikes in plasma glucose led to an immediate reduction in vascular inflammation and improved endothelial function. Recent randomized controlled trials suggest that improving postprandial dysmetabolism may also reduce the incidence of type 2 diabetes (DREAM trial) and hypertension (STOP-NIDDM trial) and slow the progression of atherosclerosis (Figure 2.7). Measures shown to improve postprandial hyperglycemia (and hypertriglyceridemia) include diet/exercise (see Table 4.4, p. 44), exenatide, rosiglitazone, pioglitazone, acarbose, nateglinide, repaglinide, ultra-fast–acting insulins, and sitagliptin.

D. **Prevention of Type 2 Diabetes.** The incidence of diabetes and prediabetes has been on a steeply rising trajectory that parallels the obesity epidemic. More than 150 million people worldwide have diabetes, and the number of cases is expected to double by the year 2025. The typical American born today has a one in three chance of developing type 2 diabetes; for Hispanics and African-Americans, the risk is one in two. Diabetes confers a level of cardiovascular risk similar to that associated with a history of prior MI and is considered a "CHD risk equivalent." (The converse is also true: over 70% of people who present with CHD have abnormal glucose metabolism [European Heart Journal 2004;25:1880-1890].) Risk factors for the development of type 2 diabetes are shown in Table 2.4. For a person diagnosed with diabetes under age 50, mean life expectancy is reduced by 12.5 to 14 years and quality of

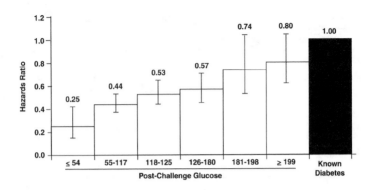

Figure 2.5. Postprandial Glucose Levels and Cardiovascular Risk

The risk of cardiovascular death increases 300% as 2-hour post-challenge glucose levels rise from 54 mg/dL to 199 mg/dL, despite the fact that these readings are all in the nondiabetic range. Hazard ratios and 95% confidence intervals for cardiovascular mortality, as assessed during 11-year follow up for 29,714 patients in the DECODE study. From: Diabetes Care 2003; 26:688-96.

life by 20 years (JAMA 2003;290:1884-90). Because of its high prevalence and grave health consequences, the prevention of type 2 diabetes has become a major focus of health care. Diet and exercise can substantially improve insulin sensitivity, lower plasma insulin levels, improve manifestations of the metabolic syndrome, and prevent/delay type 2 diabetes by up to 58%. For patients with pre-diabetes (IGT or IFG), the American Diabetes Association recommends counseling on weight loss of 5-10% of body weight and increasing moderately-intense physical activity (50-70% of maximal heart rate) to at least 150 minutes per week. For obese individuals under age 60 who are at very high risk (i.e., IGT and IFG plus other risk factors), ADA guidelines state that use of metformin may be considered (Diabetes Care 2008;31[suppl 1]:S12-S55). Rosiglitazone, metformin, acarbose, and orlistat have also been

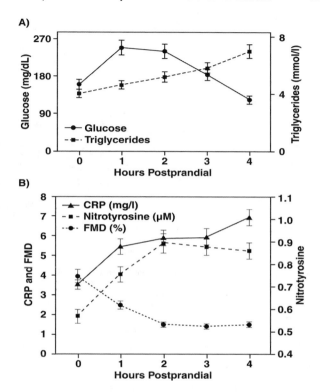

Figure 2.6. Postprandial Glucose Levels and Endothelial Function

The immediate deleterious effects of a meal containing 75 grams of glucose and 700 kcal/m^2 of whipping cream in 20 diabetic subjects. (A) Within 2-4 hours glucose and triglyceride levels double. (B) This causes immediate oxidant stress (increased nitrotyrosine levels) and vascular inflammation (increased CRP), resulting in deterioration in endothelial function (reduction in percent flow mediated dilatation, FMD). From: Circulation 2005;111:2518-24.

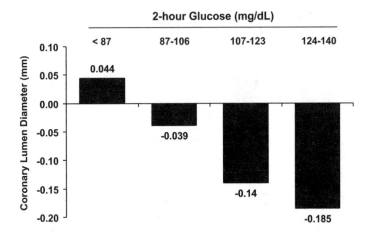

Figure 2.7. Postprandial Glucose Levels and Progression of Atherosclerosis

Angiographic coronary disease progression as measured by change in minimum coronary lumen diameter. In this cohort of patients with normal glucose tolerance as defined by a 2-hour postchallenge glucose of < 140mg/dL, the patients who showed a peak postprandial glucose of less that 87 mg/dL had coronary regression. The remaining patients had coronary progression in proportion to the rise in postprandial glucose. From: Arterioscler Thromb Vasc Biol 2006;26:189-93.

shown to reduce new diabetes in prospective randomized trials (Table 2.5). The largest and most impressive of these studies was the Diabetes REduction Assessment with ramipril and rosiglitazone Medication (DREAM) trial, which evaluated the effectiveness of rosiglitazone and/or ramipril for preventing type 2 diabetes and death in prediabetic individuals. A total of 5269 adults aged 30 years or more with IFG (mean FPG 104 mg/dL) or IGT (mean 2-hour post-challenge blood glucose 156 mg/dL) were randomized to rosiglitazone 8 mg/d or placebo in a factorial design. After three years, rosiglitazone reduced the primary endpoint—new diabetes or death—by 60% (11.6% of the rosiglitazone group versus 26.0% of the placebo group, p < 0.0001) (Figure 2.8). Additionally, 50.5% of rosiglitazone-treated patients versus 30.3% of the placebo group reverted back to normoglycemia during the course of the study (p < 0.0001). Cardiovascular event rates were similar in the two groups, except for congestive heart failure, which developed in 0.5% of the rosiglitazone group and in 0.1% of the placebo group (p = 0.01). At study end, the median fasting plasma glucose was 9 mg/dL lower and the 2-hour post-challenge blood glucose was 30 mg/dL lower in the rosiglitazone group compared to placebo. Based on these results it was estimated that rosiglitazone 8 mg/d for 3 years would prevent one in every seven people with IGT or IFG from developing diabetes (Lancet 2006;368:1096-1105).

ACE inhibitors, and angiotensin receptor blockers (ARBs) may also be useful in preventing new diabetes (Table 2.6). In a meta-analysis of post-hoc analyses of 13 randomized ACE inhibitor and ARB trials, including 90,474 patients without diabetes at baseline, risk reduction for new onset diabetes was 24% for ACE inhibitors and 23% for ARBs (overall RRR 0.77 [95% CI: 0.71-0.83]) (J Am Coll Cardiol 2005;46:821-826). The new diagnosis of diabetes was a prespecified endpoint in the VALUE trial, which compared the blood pressure effects of valsartan (ARB) versus amlodipine, a calcium channel blocker. A significant 23% decrease in new onset diabetes was seen in the valsartan treated group. In contrast, in the DREAM trial, a nonsignificant 9% reduction in new-onset diabetes was seen with ramipril 15 mg/d (N Engl J Med 2006;355:1551-62). Also, while pravastatin reduced new-onset diabetes by 30% in a post-hoc analysis of the West of Scotland study (Circulation 2001;103:357-62), simvastatin did not reduce the prespecified endpoint of new-onset diabetes in the Heart Protection Study (HPS). Additional trials will be needed to confirm these findings, and other prospective trials are underway (NAVIGATOR: valsartan and nateglinide; ACT NOW: pioglitazone). At present, no pharmacologic agent is approved for the prevention of diabetes.

Table 2.4. Risk Factors for Type 2 Diabetes

- Age ≥ 45 years
- Overweight (body mass index ≥ 25 kg/m^2*)
- First-degree relative with diabetes
- Habitual physical inactivity
- Member of a high-risk ethnic population (e.g., African American, Latino, Native American, Asian American, Pacific Islander)
- Impaired fasting glucose (IFG) or impaired glucose tolerance (IGT)
- History of gestational diabetes or delivery of a baby weighting > 9 lbs
- Hypertensive (≥ 140/90 mmHg)
- HDL cholesterol ≤ 35 mg/dL or triglyceride level ≥ 250 mg/dL
- Polycystic ovary syndrome
- History of vascular disease

* May not be correct for all ethnic groups. From: Diabetes Care 2007;30(suppl 1)

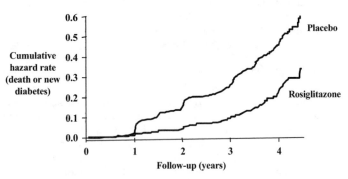

Figure 2.8. Results of the DREAM Trial

Rosiglitazone 8 mg/d for 3 years reduced by 60% the incidence of new diabetes in adults with impaired fasting glucose (IFG) or impaired glucose tolerance (IGT) (11.6% in the rosiglitazone group vs. 26% in the placebo group, RRR 60%, HR 0.40 [0.35-0.46], p < 0.0001). Reversion to normoglycemia was also significantly more likely to occur with rosiglitazone (p < 0.0001). From: Lancet 2006; 268:1096-1105.

Table 2.5. Prevention of Type 2 Diabetes: Randomized Controlled Trials in Persons with Impaired Glucose Tolerance (IGT)

Trial	No. Patients	Follow-up (years)	Risk Reduction Measure	Reduction in New Diabetes
DREAM	5269	3	Rosiglitazone Ramipril	60% 9%
Diabetes Prevention Project (DPP)	3234	2.8	Metformin Diet/exercise	31% 58%
Indian Diabetes Prevention Program	531	2.5	Metformin Diet/exercise	26% 29%
Finish Diabetes Prevention Study	522	3.2	Intensive diet/exercise	58%
Da Quing IGT & Diabetes Study	577	6	Diet/exercise	31-46%
SOS	1703	10	Bariatric surgery	70%
STOP-NIDDM	1400	3.9	Acarbose	25%
TRIPOD	266*	2.5	Troglitazone	55%
XENDOS	3304	4	Orlistat	37%

* Hispanic women with gestational diabetes mellitus

Lifestyle changes are recommended for all patients at risk for developing type 2 diabetes. No drug therapy has been approved for the prevention of new diabetes. References: DREAM: Diabetes Reduction Assessment with Ramipril and Rosiglitazone Medication (Lancet 2006;368:1096-1105); DPP: Diabetes Prevention Study (N Engl J Med 2001;344:1343-1350); Indian Diabetes Prevention Study (Diabetologia 2006;49:289-97); SOS: Swedish Obese Subjects (N Eng J Med 2004;351:2683-93); STOP-NIDDM: Study to Prevent NIDDM (Lancet 2002;359:2072-2077); TRIPOD: Troglitazone in the Prevention of Diabetes (Diabetes 2002;51:2796-2803); XENDOS: Xenical in the Prevention of Diabetes in Obese Subjects (Rev Med Liege 2002;57:617-621).

Table 2.6. Prevention of Type 2 Diabetes: Other Randomized Trials[†]

Trial	No. Patients	Follow-up (years)	Comparison	Reduction in New Diabetes
VALUE	15,245 with hypertension + ASVD or diabetes	4.2	Valsartan vs. amlodipine	23%
HOPE	9297 with ASVD or diabetes*	5	Ramipril vs. placebo	34%
ALLHAT	24,309 with hypertension + 1 cardiac risk factor	4.9	Lisinopril vs. chlorthalidone	30%
PEACE	8290 with CHD	4.8	Trandolapril vs. placebo	20%
ANBP2	6083 with hypertension	4.1	Enalapril vs. hydrochlorothiazide	33%
CAPPP	10,985 with hypertension	5	Captopril vs. diuretic/beta-blocker	15%
ASCOT	19,257 with hypertension plus ≥ 3 other risk factors	5.4	Amlodipine + perindopril vs. atenolol + diuretic	32%
LIFE	9193 with hypertension/ LVH	4.8	Losartan vs. atenolol	25%
CHARM	7601 with chronic heart failure	3.2	Candesartan vs. placebo	29%
COMET	3029 with chronic heart failure	4.8	Carvedilol vs. metoprolol	22%

ASVD = atherosclerotic vascular disease, LVH = left ventricular hypertrophy

† All are post-hoc analyses except for VALUE, where diagnosis of new diabetes was a prespecified endpoint. No drug therapy is approved for the prevention of new diabetes

* With at least 1 other cardiovascular risk factor

References: VALUE (Lancet 2004;363:2022-31); HOPE (N Engl J Med 2000;342:145-153, JAMA 2001;286:1882-5); ALLHAT (JAMA 2002;288:2981-2997, JAMA 2000;283:1967-1975); PEACE (N Engl J Med 2004;251:2058-68); ANBP2 (N Engl J Med 2003;348:583-92); CAPPP (Lancet 1999;353:611-616, Diabetes Care 2001;24:2091-2096); ASCOT (ACC meeting, March, 2005, Orlando, FL); LIFE (Lancet 2002;359:995-1003); CHARM (Lancet 2003;362:759-766); COMET (Lancet 2003;362:7-13).

Chapter 3

Overview of Treatment of Type 2 Diabetes

Once the diagnosis of diabetes has been established (Chapter 1), the medical history, physical examination, and laboratory testing (Table 3.1) are used to identify cardiovascular risk factors and target organ damage:

- *Cardiovascular risk factors*: hypertension, dyslipidemia, sedentary lifestyle, overweight/obesity, tobacco use, atherogenic diet
- *Cardiovascular disease:* angina, prior MI or coronary revascularization, heart failure, left ventricular hypertrophy
- *Cerebrovascular disease:* carotid bruit, transient ischemic attack, stroke
- *Retinopathy:* microaneurysms, hard exudates, macular edema, soft exudates (retinal infarcts), neovascularization, vitreous hemorrhage, retinal detachment, macular ischemia, rubeosis iritis, diabeticorum acute glaucoma
- *Nephropathy:* increased serum creatinine, micro/macroalbuminuria
- *Peripheral artery disease:* claudication, aneurysm, absence of peripheral pulses, foot ulcers, loss of hair growth, shiny thin skin
- *Neuropathy:* altered light touch/pain/vibration, orthostatic hypotension, fixed heart rate, gastroparesis, urinary retention, diabetic diarrhea, erectile impotence, excessive sweating, small pupils, muscle weakness, neuropathic pain, foot ulcers, interosseous muscle wasting

Glycemic Control

Epidemiologic analysis from the United Kingdom Prospective Diabetes Study (UKPDS) Group demonstrated a continuous relationship between baseline glycemia and the risk of vascular complications: each 1% decrease in HbA_{1c} was associated with a 35% reduction in microvascular complications, a 25% reduction in diabetes-related deaths, an 18% reduction in MI, and a 7% reduction in all-cause mortality. Compared to patients treated conservatively with diet in UKPDS (mean HbA_{1c} 7.9%), intensive glycemic therapy with either a sulfonylurea or insulin (mean HbA_{1c} 7%) was

Table 3.1. Clinical Evaluation of Type 2 Diabetes

Medical History
- Symptoms, laboratory tests, other results related to the diagnosis of diabetes
- Prior HbA$_{1c}$ records and details of previous and current treatment programs (medications, meal plan, results of glucose monitoring and patients' use of data)
- Eating patterns, nutritional status, and weight history; growth and development in children and adolescents; exercise history
- Frequency, severity, cause of acute complications (e.g., ketoacidosis, hypoglycemia)
- Prior or current infections (e.g., skin, foot, dental, genitourinary)
- Symptoms and treatment of complication of diabetes (eye, kidney, nerve, heart, peripheral vascular, bladder, GI, foot, cerebrovascular)
- Other medications that may affect blood glucose levels
- Risk factors for atherosclerosis (smoking, hypertension, overweight/obesity, dyslipidemia, sedentary lifestyle, family history)
- History and treatment of other conditions, including endocrine and eating disorders
- Family history of diabetes and other endocrine disorders
- Lifestyle, cultural, psychosocial, educational, and economic factors that might influence the management of diabetes
- Tobacco, alcohol, controlled substance use
- Contraception and reproductive/sexual history

Physical Examination
- Height, weight, waist circumference measurements, BMI calculation
- Blood pressure (including orthostatic) measurements
- Funduscopic, oral, thyroid, cardiac, hand/finger examinations
- Neurological exam, including vibration sense (tuning fork)/fine sensation (monofilament)
- Abdominal examination (e.g., for hepatomegaly); skin examination (for acanthosis nigricans and insulin-injection sites); evaluation of pulses by palpation/auscultation
- Signs of diseases that can cause secondary diabetes (e.g., hemochromatosis, pancreatic disease, Cushing's disease)

Laboratory Evaluation
- HbA$_{1c}$
- Fasting total/LDL/HDL cholesterol and triglycerides
- Test for microalbuminuria; urinalysis for ketones, protein, sediment
- Serum creatinine in adults (in children if proteinuria is present)
- Thyroid-stimulating hormone (TSH) if clinically indicated
- Bone density in adults > 50 years old (diabetes is a risk factor for osteoporosis)
- Electrocardiogram in adults

Referrals
- Eye exam; family planning for women of reproductive age; diabetes educator, if not provided by physician or staff; behavioral specialist; foot specialist; dietician; others

Adapted from: The American Diabetes Association. Diabetes Care 2008;31(suppl 1):S12-S55.

associated with a highly significant 25% reduction in microvascular complications and a 16% reduction in MI and death at 10 years (p = 0.052). The Norfolk Epic Study showed that for each 1% HbA_{1c} increase above 5% and 7%, cardiac events increased by 26% and 40%, respectively.

A. **Goals of Therapy.** Diabetes treatment goals differ somewhat between the American Diabetes Association (ADA), the American Association of Clinical Endocrinologists/American College of Endocrinology (AACE/ACE), and the International Diabetes Federation (Table 3.2). (The ADA recommendation is based on the results of DCCT, a type 1 diabetes study [p. 159]; the AACE/ACE recommendation is based on the results of UKPDS, a type 2 study [p. 162]). In general, efforts should be made to reduce HbA_{1c} to the lowest possible level at which frequent or severe hypoglycemic episodes do not occur. Unlike patients with type 1 diabetes, in most patients with type 2 diabetes, HbA_{1c} levels between 6-7% are readily achieved. This is especially the case in the earlier stages

Table 3.2. Treatment Targets for Adults with Diabetes

	Normal	ADA Target	AACE/ACE Target
Glycemic control			
HbA_{1c} (%)*	< 5.8	< 7.0	< 6.5
Plasma glucose			
preprandial	< 100	70-130	< 110
postprandial	< 140[†]	< 180[¶]	< 140[†]
Blood pressure (mmHg)	< 120/80	< 130/80	–
Lipids (mg/dL)			
LDL	< 130	< 100[‡]	–
Triglycerides[‡]	< 150	< 150[‡]	–
HDL	> 40	> 40	–

AACE/ACE = American Association of Clinical Endocrinologists/American College of Endocrinology (Endocr Pract 2002;8[suppl 1]:5-11), ADA = American Diabetes Association (Diabetes Care 2008;31[suppl 1]:S12-S55)

* Referenced to a nondiabetic range of 4.0-6.0% using a DCCT-based assay
† 2-hour postprandial
¶ Peak postprandial
‡ For diabetic patients with established CHD or other clinical forms of atherosclerosis, it is reasonable to treat to an optional LDL-C < 70 mg/dL and, if triglycerides ≥ 200 mg/dL, to an optional non–HDL-C < 100 mg/dL (Circulation 2004;110:227-239, Circulation 2006;113:2363-2372) (also see Chapter 7)

of type 2 diabetes when endogenous insulin production is still high, particularly if drugs that do not cause hypoglycemia are utilized (metformin, TZDs, alpha-glucosidase inhibitors, DPP-4 inhibitors) (Chapter 5). The risks and benefits of intensive glycemic control for patients with type 2 diabetes are described in Chapter 5.

B. **Assessment of Glycemic Control.** Monitoring of glycemic status by patients and physicians is essential to diabetes management. Results are used to evaluate the effectiveness of therapy and to guide changes in diet, exercise, and medications.

   1. **Self-monitoring of blood glucose.** Self-monitoring of blood glucose allows rapid and precise adjustments in treatment and monitoring/prevention of asymptomatic hypoglycemia. It also improves compliance, by allowing patients to participate in their own care, and reinforces the importance of diet and exercise.

   Most individuals with type 1 diabetes and pregnant females treated with insulin will require self-monitoring, ideally on a daily basis before meals and bedtime, two hours after main meals, during the night, and when symptoms of hypoglycemia occur. Equipment that continuously monitors glucose concentrations in interstitial fluid and warns of hypoglycemia is being utilized to achieve even better control than with traditional self-monitoring; however, standardization with traditional self-monitoring equipment is required on a twice daily basis.

   For persons with type 2 diabetes, the frequency of self-monitoring is based on the treatment regimen and the stability of glucose measurements, although self-monitoring in type 2 diabetic patients who do not require insulin has never been proven to improve glycemic control. More frequent monitoring is recommended for type 2 diabetic patients who are receiving insulin or insulin secretagogues and for those not at glycemic goal. Most patients should be initially instructed to record morning and pre-dinner glucose levels. As the antidiabetic regimen is intensified and glycemic targets are approached, patients should begin checking preprandial and 2-hour postprandial glucose levels with at least one meal per day (ideally with every meal). This will allow pre- and postprandial glucose patterns to emerge over 1-2 weeks so that drug therapy can be refined. It is important to teach patients proper monitoring technique and how to adjust their diet, exercise, and medications based on blood glucose measurements, though self-monitoring in the type 2 patient who does not need insulin has never been proven to improve glycemic control. Patients should also be reminded to check their meter and strips using the control solution at least once a month or whenever they open a new bottle of strips, whichever is sooner. Proper monitoring technique should be periodically confirmed.

2. **Hemoglobin A_{1c}.** Hemoglobin is continuously glycated during the 120-day life span of the erythrocyte. Hemoglobin A_{1c} (HbA$_{1c}$), the major glycated subfraction, has provided a tool to monitor the 6-week to 3-month average of a patient's glucose control. (The cumulative amount of HbA$_{1c}$ in an erythrocyte is directly proportional to the time-averaged concentration of glucose in the bloodstream and is not affected by acute changes in blood glucose or recent food intake.) Ideal HbA$_{1c}$ levels are $\leq 5.0\%$, while levels $> 6.0\%$ are virtually diagnostic of diabetes. HbA$_{1c}$ levels may be artificially low in uremia, hemoglobinopathy, pregnancy, blood transfusion, and hemolytic anemia. For patients with uremia or hemoglobinopathy, glycated serum protein, which reflects the degree of glucose binding to serum protein (mainly albumin), or fructosamine can be used as an index of glycemic control over the previous 4-8 weeks and 2-4 weeks, respectively. The fructosamine level may be utilized in pregnancy, since better outcomes for the pregnancy and offspring are associated with earlier detection and management of changes in glycemic control. The American Diabetes Association recommends HbA$_{1c}$ testing every 3 months in patients whose therapy has changed or who have not yet met treatment goals and at least twice yearly in patients with stable glycemic control meeting target goals. The assay for HbA$_{1c}$ has not yet been standardized, and each lab reports a different reference range depending on the assay used. In the U.S., the NGSP has succeeded in standardizing approximately 95% of the laboratories, with results certified as "traceable to the DCCT A_{1C} assay." However, the sensitivity, specificity, and accuracy of the HbA$_{1c}$ test is still not sufficient to allow the assay to be used to diagnose diabetes, and in

many countries, HbA$_{1c}$ assays are not widely available. HbA$_{1c}$ can also be used to confirm the accuracy of self-reported blood glucose measurements (Table 3.3).

C. **Types of Therapy.** Therapeutic lifestyle changes—medical nutritional therapy, exercise, weight control, smoking cessation—are mandatory to optimize glycemic control and reduce cardiovascular risk (Chapter 4). Five functional classes of oral pharmacologic agents are available for the treatment of type 2 diabetes: biguanides, thiazolidinediones (TZDs), alpha-glucosidase inhibitors, insulin secretagogues, and DPP-4 inhibitors (Chapter 5). In addition there are three functional classes of subcutaneous injectable agents: insulin, incretin mimetics (exenatide), and amylin mimetics (pramlintide). Insulin therapy is usually reserved for type 2 diabetic patients with inadequate glycemic control despite lifestyle changes and maximized oral combination therapy. Special therapeutic considerations for individuals with advanced age, acute MI, gestational diabetes, or severe/frequent hypoglycemic episodes are described in Chapter 5.

Table 3.3. Correlation Between HbA$_{1c}$ with Mean Plasma Glucose Levels

	Mean plasma glucose	
HbA$_{1c}$	mg/dL	mmol/L
12	345	19.5
11	310	17.5
10	275	15.5
9	240	13.5
8	205	11.5
7	170	9.5
6	135	7.5

From: Standards of Medical Care in Diabetes. The American Diabetes Association. Diabetes Care 2008;31(suppl 1):S12-S55.

Other Therapeutic Considerations

Control of hypertension and dyslipidemia, smoking cessation, increased physical activity, weight control, and use of antiplatelet therapy, ACE inhibitors or ARBs, beta blockers, and statins reduce cardiovascular events in type 2 diabetes (Chapters 7-9). Treatment targets for blood pressure and lipids are shown in Table 3.2. Annual influenza vaccine is recommended for all individuals > 6 months of age, and pneumococcal vaccine is recommended for adult diabetic patients, with one-time revaccination in some (individuals previously immunized at < 65 years of age who are now > 64 years of age and who received vaccine > 5 years ago; nephrotic syndrome; chronic renal disease; or organ transplantation) (Diabetes Care 2005;28[suppl 1]:S4-S36). Use of shingles vaccine should be considered for patient over age 60 with diabetes. Screening for and early treatment of atherosclerotic vascular disease, retinopathy, nephropathy, distal symmetrical polyneuropathy, and foot ulcers are mandatory in all patients (Chapter 6). Early psychosocial assessment is recommended to identify patients at risk for medical noncompliance and depression (pp. 60-62).

Patient Education

Many diabetic individuals are unaware that they are at increased risk of heart attack and stroke and are unable to identify more than one early warning sign of these conditions. Also, more than 50% of patients discontinue hypertension, diabetes, and dyslipidemia medications without informing their physician. All persons with diabetes should be educated about the silent nature of their disease, the risks if left untreated, proper technique for self-monitoring of blood glucose, and the method for adjusting diet, activity, and medications based on blood glucose measurments. Adherence to diabetes therapy can also be improved by challenging patients to play an active role in their disease—recording blood glucose at home, reporting side effects, involving their families, challenging them to reach and maintain the therapeutic goal. Hypertensive patients should be encouraged to record and report their blood pressure prior to their morning drug dose (to ensure protection against the surge in blood pressure upon awakening) and in the early evening (to ensure coverage throughout the day). Compliance measures should be reinforced at every visit, including the importance of continuing statins and hypertension and diabetes medications.

Chapter 4

Therapeutic Lifestyle Changes

Diet modification, weight control, and increased physical activity are important therapeutic lifestyle changes for all persons with diabetes, prediabetes, or the metabolic syndrome. For patients requiring pharmacologic therapy for diabetes, hypertension or dyslipidemia, drugs should be added to, not substituted for, diet modification and other lifestyle changes.

Medical Nutritional Therapy

Medical nutritional therapy (MNT) is a cornerstone to therapy for patients with type 2 diabetes. MNT helps to achieve and maintain glycemic control, desirable body weight, improved lipid profile, and lowered blood pressure, thus reducing cardiovascular risk. A coordinated team approach, including a registered dietician (team leader), physician, nurse and patient, will optimize implementation of and compliance with MNT. Nutritional recommendations from the American Diabetes Association and National Cholesterol Education Program – Adult Treatment Panel III are shown in Tables 4.1 and 4.2). Table 4.3 lists dietary measures to lower LDL cholesterol.

Table 4.1. Nutritional Recommendations for Type 2 Diabetes

Food Composition	Recommendation
Total fat *Saturated fat** *Polyunsaturated fat* *Monounsaturated fat*	25-35% of total calories < 7% of total calories Up to 10% of total calories‡ Up to 20% of total calories
Carbohydrates	40-50% of total calories†
Fiber	25-40 gm/d
Protein	15-20% of total calories¶
Cholesterol	< 200 mg/d
Total calories	Sufficient to maintain desirable body weight

*   Trans fats also raise LDL cholesterol and should be avoided

† Most as complex carbohydrates from vegetables, fruits, and whole grains (low glycemic index). Monitoring carbohydrate intake is crucial for achieving glycemic control. Moderate use of sugar alcohols and non-nutritive sweeteners is safe

‡ Two or more servings of fish (non-fried) per week provide omega-3 polyunsaturated fatty acids and is recommended

¶ For diabetic patients with early or late stage chronic renal disease, protein intake should be restricted to 0.8-1.0 gm/kg body weight/day and 0.8 gm/kg body weight/day, respectively

Adapted from: National Cholesterol Education Program ATP III (Circulation 2002;106:3145-3421); Nutritional Recommendations and Interventions for Diabetes: The American Diabetes Association (Diabetes Care 2008;31[suppl 1]:S61-S78)

Table 4.2. Components of Medical Nutritional Therapy

Component	Evidence	Recommendations
Total fat	Polyunsaturated and monounsaturated fats do not raise LDL cholesterol when substituted for carbohydrates in the diet.	It is not necessary to restrict total fat intake provided saturated fats and trans fats are minimized.
Saturated fats	High intakes of saturated fats raise LDL cholesterol and are associated with high population rates of CHD. Reduction in intake of saturated fats reduces CHD risk.	A therapeutic diet to maximize LDL-lowering should contain < 7% of total calories as saturated fats.
Trans fats	Trans fats raise LDL cholesterol. Prospective studies support an association between higher intakes of trans fats and CHD. Trans fats comprise 2% of the average American diet; eliminating these fats from diet could reduce cardiovascular events up to 50%.	Intakes of trans fats should be kept low. Extra virgin olive oil, soft margarine, and trans fat-free margarine are encouraged instead of butter, stick margarine, and shortening.
Polyunsaturated fats	Linoleic acid and linolenic polyunsaturated fat reduce LDL cholesterol levels when substituted for saturated fats. Clinical trials indicate that substitution of polyunsaturated fats for saturated fats reduces risk for CHD.	Polyunsaturated fats can replace saturated fat. Most polyunsaturated fats should be derived from nuts, avocados, olive and canola oils. Intake can range up to 10% of total calories.

Table 4.2. Components of Medical Nutritional Therapy (cont'd)

Component	Evidence	Recommendations
Mono-unsaturated fats	Monounsaturated fats lower LDL cholesterol relative to saturated fatty acids but do not lower HDL cholesterol or raise triglycerides. Diets rich in monounsaturated fats provided by plant sources and rich in fruits, vegetables, and whole grains and low in saturated fats decrease CHD risk.	Monounsaturated fats are one form of unsaturated fatty acid that can replace saturated fats. Intake can range up to 20% of total calories. Most monounsaturated fats should be derived from vegetable sources, including avocados, nuts, peanuts, olive oil, canola oil.
Cholesterol	High intakes of dietary cholesterol raise LDL cholesterol and the risk for CHD. Reducing intakes from high to low decreases LDL cholesterol.	Less than 200 mg per day of cholesterol should be consumed in the TLC Diet to maximize LDL cholesterol lowering.
Carbohydrates	When carbohydrate is substituted for saturated fats, LDL cholesterol falls. However, very high intakes of carbohydrate (>60% of total calories) lower HDL cholesterol and raise triglycerides and glycemic index. Diabetics are especially sensitive to excessive carbohydrate intake (particularly in the form of sugar and starches), which typically results in worsening insulin resistance.	Monitoring carbohydrate intake is crucial for achieving glycemic control. Daily intake should be limited to ≤ 40-50% of total calories. Most carbohydrates should come from low glycemic index vegetables, fruits, legumes, and whole grains. Sugar alcohols and non-nutritive sweeteners when used in moderation are safe.

Table 4.2. Components of Medical Nutritional Therapy (cont'd)

Component	Evidence	Recommendations
Protein	Substituting vegetable protein (nuts, soy foods, legumes, etc.) for animal protein has been reported to lower LDL cholesterol. Lean animal protein (nonfat dairy, whey protein, egg whites, skinless poultry, fish, etc.) improves satiety and slows gastric emptying and can thereby help improve excess body weight and hyperglycemia.	Protein intake should constitute ~ 15-25% of total calories. Plant sources of protein include legumes, dry beans, nuts, and to a lesser extent, grain products and vegetables, which are low in saturated fats/cholesterol. Animal sources of protein lower in saturated fat/cholesterol include fat-free/low-fat dairy, egg whites, fish, skinless poultry, lean meats.

Adapted from: National Cholesterol Education Program ATP III Report. Circulation 2002;106:3145-3421; Nutritional Recommendations and Interventions for Diabetes: The American Diabetes Association (Diabetes Care 2008;31[suppl 1]:S61-S78)

Table 4.3. Dietary Options for LDL-Lowering and Cardiovascular Risk Reduction: Recommendations from NCEP-ATP III

Measure	Evidence Statement*	Comments
Increasing viscous fiber in the diet	5-10 gm/d of viscous fiber reduces LDL cholesterol levels by ~ 5%.	Dietary viscous fiber is a therapeutic option to enhance LDL-lowering.
Plant stanols/sterols	Intakes of 1.5-3 gm/d of plant stanol/sterol esters reduce LDL cholesterol by 6-15%.	Plant stanol/sterol esters are a therapeutic option to enhance LDL-lowering.
Soy protein	High intakes of soy protein can lower LDL cholesterol up to 5%, especially when it replaces animal food products.	Food sources containing soy protein are acceptable as replacements for animal food products containing animal fats.

Table 4.3. Dietary Options for LDL-Lowering and Cardiovascular Risk Reduction: Recommendations from NCEP-ATP III (cont'd)

Measure	Evidence Statement*	Comments
n-3 (omega-3) polyunsaturated fatty acids	Higher intakes of n-3 fatty acids may reduce coronary events/mortality, lower triglycerides by 25-50%, and raise HDL by 8%.	Patients with diabetes or CHD should consume at least 500-1000 mg of EPA + DHA per day, either from fatty fish (2-4 times per week) or fish oil capsules (2-3 capsules per day).
Folic acid and vitamins B_6 and B_{12}	There are no randomized trials to show that dietary/vitamin lowering of homocysteine will reduce CHD risk.	ATP III endorses the Institute of Medicine RDA for dietary folate (400 mcg/d).
Antioxidants	Clinical trials have failed to show antioxidant supplements reduce CHD risk. Diets naturally high in antioxidants (fruits, vegetables, green tea, red wine) do appear to confer cardiovascular protection.	The Institute of Medicine's RDAs for dietary antioxidants are recommended (vitamin C: 75 mg and 90 mg/d for women and men; vitamin E: 15 IU/d).
Low to moderate alcohol intake	Low to moderate alcohol intake in middle-aged/older adults may reduce CHD risk. High intakes of alcohol produce multiple adverse effects.	Alcohol should be limited to not more than 2 drinks per day for men and not more than 1 drink per day for women. A drink is defined as 5.5 oz. wine, 12 oz. beer, or 1.5 oz. 80-proof whiskey.
Dietary sodium, potassium, calcium, and magnesium	Lower sodium intake lowers blood pressure or prevents its rise. Higher dietary intakes of potassium, magnesium and calcium can reduce blood pressure.	ATP III supports JNC 7 recommendation of a sodium intake of < 2.4 gm/d sodium or 6.4 gm/d sodium chloride and adequate intakes of dietary potassium (~ 90 mmol/day), calcium, and magnesium.

Table 4.3. Dietary Options for LDL-Lowering and Cardiovascular Risk Reduction: Recommendations from NCEP-ATP III (cont'd)

Measure	Evidence Statement*	Comments
Herbal or botanical dietary supplements	Trial data are not available to support herbal/botanical supplements in the prevention or treatment of heart disease. Ephedrine-containing products can cause fatal cardiovascular complications and should not be used.	ATP III does not recommend use of herbal/botanical supplements to reduce CHD risk. Patients should be asked if such products are being used because of potential drug interactions.
High protein, high total fat and saturated fat weight loss regimens	These diets (like the Atkins Diet) have not been shown in controlled trials to improve cardiovascular health, and their nutrient composition is potentially atherogenic.	These regimens are not recommended for weight reduction in clinical practice.

Adapted from: National Cholesterol Education Program Adult Treatment Panel III Report. Circulation 2002;106:3145-3421.

Dietary Strategies To Improve Postprandial Dysmetabolism and Cardiovascular Health

Epidemiological data consistently demonstrate that postprandial hyperglycemia is an independent predictor of future cardiovascular events (Figure 2.5) and atherosclerosis progression (Figure 2.7). The cardiovascular toxicity of postprandial hyperglycemia/hyperlipemia (dysmetabolism) appears to be mediated by oxidant stress, which is directly proportional to glucose and lipid excursion after a meal. This transient increase in free radical formation acutely triggers inflammation, endothelial dysfunction, hypercoagulability, sympathetic hyperactivity, and a cascade of other atherogenic changes (Figure 2.6). Steps to improve postprandial dysmetabolism include consumption of a Mediterranean-style diet (see next section), increased physical activity, and maintaining ideal body weight (Table 4.4).

Table 4.4. Steps to Improve Postprandial Glucose and Triglycerides

- Choose high-fiber, low glycemic index carbohydrates such as whole grains, legumes, vegetables and fruits

- Eat lean protein at all 3 meals

- Consume nuts on a daily basis, about 1 handful (with a closed fist). Eat with vegetables, berries or other fruits, or grains

- Eat a salad of leafy greens with vinegar and virgin olive oil dressing on a daily basis

- Avoid highly processed foods and drinks, especially those with sugar, high-fructose corn syrup, white flour, or trans fats

- Keep serving sizes modest

- Consider consuming 1 alcoholic drink before or with the evening meal

- Avoid being overweight or obese; maintain a waist circumference less than one-half of height in inches

- Obtain 30 minutes or more of daily physical activity of at least moderate intensity

Source: J Am Coll Cardiol 2008;51:249-55.

Mediterranean-Style Diet

A. **Lyon Heart Study**. Increasing evidence suggests that a Mediterranean-style diet emphasizing consumption of monounsaturated and omega-3 fatty acids can play an important role in the prevention of atherothrombotic vascular disease. The Lyon Diet Heart Study randomized 605 patients post-MI to a Mediterranean diet providing increased levels of alpha-linolenic acid (from olive oil and canola oil) or usual dietary instruction. Patients in the Mediterranean diet group were instructed to consume more fish, fruit, and vegetables; eat less meat; and use canola-based margarine and olive oil as a fat source. After 27 months, patients on the Mediterranean diet showed a 70% reduction in all-cause mortality (p = 0.03). The rate of cardiovascular death and nonfatal MI was 1.32 per 100 patient years in the treated group compared to 5.55 per 100 patient years in the control group (p = 0.001) (Lancet 1994;343:1454-9). Risk reduction correlated with best increased omega-3 intake in the treatment group. Benefits were maintained at 4 years (Circulation 1999;99:779-85).

B. **Other Studies.** The GISSI Prevention study randomized 11,324 Italian men and women (who presumably were eating a Mediterranean diet) with MI within the preceding 3 months to omega-3 fatty acid capsules (850-882 mg/d), vitamin E (300 mg/d), both, or neither. After 3.5 years, the omega-3 fatty acid group had a significant 20% reduction in all-cause mortality and 45% reduction in sudden cardiac death (Lancet 1999;354:447-55). In the Diet and Reinfarction Trial (DART), 2033 men with prior MI were randomized to receive different types of dietary advice to prevent another MI. After 2 years, the group told to increase their omega-3 fatty acid intake by eating oily fish (e.g., salmon, herring, mackerel) at least twice weekly had a 29% reduction in overall mortality (p < 0.05) (Lancet 1989;2:757-61). Results from the Nurses' Health Study, which examined the risk for CHD in 84,688 previously healthy women, found that higher consumption of fish and omega-3 fatty acids reduced the risk for cardiac death by up to 45% at 16 years (JAMA 2002;287:1815-1821). Furthermore, there was an inverse relationship between fish/omega-3 fatty acid intake and thrombotic stroke. Compared to women who ate fish < 1 time/month, relative risk reductions for women who ate fish 1-3 times/month, 1 time/week, 2-4 times/week, and ≥ 5 times/week were 0.93, 0.78, 0.73, and 0.48, respectively (JAMA 2001;285:304-312). Fish consumption 1-3 times per week also reduced ischemic stroke in men in the Health Professional Follow-up Study (JAMA 2002;288:3130-6). Omega-3 fatty acids from fish oil supplements have been shown to incorporate into atherosclerotic plaque and induce changes that enhance plaque stability (Atherosclerosis 2006;7(supl):160,T$_u$-W20:3,abst; Lancet 2003;361:477-85), and adherence to a Mediterranean diet lowers levels of inflammatory/coagulation markers (C-reactive protein, WBC count, interleukin-6, homocysteine, fibrinogen) (J Am Coll Cardiol 2004;44:152-8). Recent analysis of the National Institutes of Health (formerly AARP) Diet and Health Study, the largest study to evaluate the effect of a Mediterranean diet in a US population, reported a 20%

reduction in death or cancer (45% in smokers) associated with this diet (Arch Int Med 2007;167:2461-68). The PREDIMED study, currently in progress, is randomizing approximately 9000 patients to a Mediterranean diet (supplemented with virgin olive oil or mixed nuts) or to a low-fat diet to evaluate their impact on the primary prevention of cardiovascular events. Preliminary data at 3 months (full study to be completed in 2010) indicate beneficial effects for the Mediterranean diet on mean plasma glucose levels, systolic blood pressure, total-cholesterol/HDL-C ratio (Ann Intern Med 2006;145:1-11), and oxidized LDL-C concentrations (presented at the European Atherosclerosis Society 76th Congress; Helsinki, Finland, June, 2007). These studies suggest that the type of fat, not only the amount, can affect cardiovascular health.

C. Recommendations. Diet modification should be recommended as part of a comprehensive program to reduce vascular risk. Suggested diets are the TLC diet or a Mediterranean-style diet (Tables 4.5, 4.6).

Table 4.5. Basic Components of a Mediterranean Diet

Component	Benefits
Omega-3–rich[1] fish ≥ 2 times per week or omega-3 supplements[2]	Reduces all-cause mortality and sudden cardiac death post-MI; lowers triglycerides (high doses) and blood pressure; anti-inflammatory effects; boosts the immune system; may help prevent arthritis, depression, Alzheimer's disease.
Monounsaturated and polyunsaturated fats (olive, flaxseed, canola oils; avocados, nuts, seeds)	Do not increase LDL cholesterol or decrease HDL cholesterol (unlike high saturated fat or high intake of refined carbohydrate). "Metabolically neutral" calorie source for people with insulin resistance. Particularly effective when substituted for high glycemic load carbohydrates.
Fresh fruit and vegetables (9-12 servings per day); use wide variety	High concentrations of vitamins, minerals, fiber, and phytochemicals[3] help prevent heart disease, stroke, Alzheimer's disease, and many types of cancer (colon, stomach, prostate, pancreatic). Minimize high glycemic load fruit (e.g., bananas) and potatoes. Choose deeply pigmented, brighter colored produce.

Table 4.5. Basic Components of a Mediterranean Diet (cont'd)

Component	Benefits
Vegetable protein from nuts and beans frequently	Lowers LDL cholesterol; improves digestion; may reduce CHD and certain cancers. Nuts are an excellent source of protein, monounsaturated fat, fiber, and minerals. Beans (legumes) contain high-quality protein, fiber, potassium, and folic acid.[4]
Limit saturated fats to < 10-20 grams per day	Saturated fats increase LDL cholesterol, promote atherosclerosis, and increase the risk of CHD and stroke. Saturated fats are also linked to certain cancers.
Avoid trans fats	Trans fats are manufactured from vegetable oils and are used to enhance the taste and extend the shelf-life of fast foods, French fries, packaged snacks, commercial baked goods, and most margarines. Trans fats may be more atherogenic than saturated fats. Instruct patients to avoid foods with "hydrogenated" or "partially hydrogenated" vegetable oil—these contain trans fats.
Increase dietary to fiber to 25-40 grams per day	Lowers LDL cholesterol; improves insulin resistance; reduces the risk of heart disease and diabetes; protects against colon cancer and possibly breast cancer, irritable bowel syndrome, diverticulitis, and hemorrhoids; prevents constipation.
At least one source of high-quality protein with every meal	Produces longer-lasting satiety (reduces hunger and cravings and slows absorption of high carbohydrate meals); maintains muscle mass and bone strength. Lack of protein increases the risk of breast cancer, diabetes, and osteoporosis.

1. The typical American diet consists of an unhealthy ratio (> 15:1) of omega-6:omega-3 essential fatty acids, favoring excessive production of proinflammatory, prothrombotic, and vasoconstrictive mediators of the arachidonic acid cascade (e.g., leukotrienes, thromboxane). Increasing consumption of omega-3 essential fatty acids helps regulate inflammation, thrombogenicity, arrhythmogenicity, and vascular tone.
2. Omega-3 supplements (500-1000 mg of EPA + DHA daily) should be considered for patients with documented CHD or diabetes, especially if risk factors for sudden death are present (LV dysfunction, LVH, ventricular dysrhythmias). Dose for secondary prevention is ≥ 1000 mg EPA + DHA per day (obtainable with ~ 3 gm of standard fish oil concentrate).
3. Phytonutrients are naturally occurring chemicals found in plants—many of them plant pigments—that act as free radical scavengers and protease inhibitors, among others. Examples include lycopene, beta-carotene, indoles, thiocyanates, lutein, resveratrol, ellagic acid, genistein, flavones, anthocyanidins, and allium.
4. Folic acid lowers levels of homocysteine, a by-product of methionine metabolism associated with atherosclerosis.

Table 4.6. How to Incorporate a Mediterranean Diet into Daily Living

Step	Choose	Go Easy On	Avoid
Eat omega-3 rich food at least 2 times per week	Salmon, trout, herring, water-packed tuna, sardines, mackerel, flaxseed, spinach, purslane, fish oil supplements	Raw shellfish (due to danger of infection risk, including hepatitis A and B)	Deep-fried fish, fish sticks, fish from seriously contaminated water
Switch vegetable oils	Extra-virgin cold pressed olive oil or canola oil (check the label), flaxseed oil, mayonnaise made from olive oil or canola oil	High-oleic safflower, sunflower, or soybean oil	Corn oil, safflower oil, sunflower oil, palm oil, peanut oil, other oils, mayonnaise not from olive oil/canola oil or sweet syrups
Load up on fresh fruit and vegetables	Fresh fruit: 3-5 daily. Fresh vegetables: 4-6 daily. Use a wide variety	Fruit juice (no more than 1-2 cups per day), dried fruit, canned fruit, bananas, potatoes	Vegetables or fruit prepared in heavy cream sauces or butter
Add nuts and beans frequently	Soybeans, kidney beans, lentils, navy beans, split peas, other beans, nuts of all kinds	Heavily salted or sugared nuts	Stale or rancid nuts
Limit saturated fats to 10-20 grams per day; eat at least one source of high-quality protein with every meal	Fish, lean fresh meat with fat trimmed off, chicken and turkey without skin, nonfat or lowfat dairy products (whey protein, skim milk, yogurt, low-fat cottage cheese), dark chocolate, egg whites or egg substitute, omega-3–enriched eggs	Processed lowfat meats (bologna, salami, other luncheon meats), 2% milk, "lite" cream cheese, part-skim mozzarella cheese, milk chocolate, egg yolks (3-4 per week)	Prime-grade fatty cuts of meat, goose, duck, organ meats (liver, kidneys), full-fat processed meats, hot dogs, sausages, bacon, whole milk, cream, full-fat cheeses, cream cheese, sour cream, ice cream

Table 4.6. How to Incorporate a Mediterranean Diet into Daily Living

Step	Choose	Go Easy On	Avoid
Avoid trans fats	Stanol-enriched margarine (Benecol, Take Control), natural peanut butter, almond butter	Commercial peanut butter, water crackers and other crackers that contain no fat, bagels	Fast food, French fries and other deep-fried food, chips and other packaged snacks, most commercial baked goods, most margarines
Add more fiber; aim for 20-40 grams per day	Whole grains, oats, brown rice, wild rice, barley and wheat, whole grain versions of bread, pasta, bagels	Pasta, white rice, potatoes, plain bagels, dinner rolls, egg noodles	Sweetened cereals, white bread, crackers, table sugar, honey, syrup, candy, highly processed foods, especially those with white flour/sugar
Drink at least 64 ounces of water per day	Drink 8 glasses of pure, non-chlorinated water per day. Additional drinks: skim milk (up to 3 glasses); tea, especially green tea (up to 4 cups); decaffeinated coffee	Coffee (regular), 1% or 2% milk, fruit juice, sports drinks, diet soft drinks, alcohol (no more than 1 drink daily for women or 2 drinks daily for men)	Sugared soft drinks, milkshakes, excess alcohol, artificially sweetened fruit juices

Physical Activity

A. **Overview.** Physical inactivity increases the risk of heart disease and stroke as much as cigarette smoking, yet more than 70% of adults get little or no exercise. All patients should be encouraged to optimally obtain 30-45 minutes of aerobic activity on most days of the week. Regular exercise that increases heart rate to 60-80% of maximal peak heart rate for 30 minutes on all or most days of the week reduces the risk of MI and stroke by 50% and the risk of death post-MI by 25%. It also improves insulin resistance and type 2 diabetes (lowers HbA_{1c} by 10-20%); lowers post-prandial glucose by up to 25-50%, raises HDL cholesterol levels by up to 30%; prevents/improves hypertension, obesity, anxiety, and depression; helps smokers quit; and improves functional capacity in patients with congestive heart failure or claudication from peripheral arterial disease. Noncardiac benefits include a lower risk of cancer (colon, prostate, breast) and salutary effects on osteoporosis, arthritis, constipation, mood, insomnia, and postmenopausal symptoms. Physical activity can also delay or prevent type 2 diabetes (Chapter 2).

B. **Amount of Exercise.** The American Diabetes Association recommends a minimum of 150 minutes per week of moderately-intense (50-70% of maximal heart rate), along with resistance training 3 times per week (Diabetes Care 2008;31[suppl 1]:S12-S55). Traditionally, exercise programs have focused exclusively on aerobic activities such as walking, running, cycling, and swimming. Recent data suggest that a strength (weight) training program is an important supplement to aerobic exercise, increasing muscle mass (which increases metabolic rate), improving insulin sensitivity, and helping maintain bone and muscular strength to prevent injuries and disability. Stretching exercises (e.g., yoga) are also beneficial. Physical activity does not need to be performed in a traditional structured exercise program to provide health benefits, and a lifestyle-based exercise program incorporating physical activity into daily living is effective at improving risk factors, weight, and long-term cardiovascular prognosis (JAMA 1999;281:327-34). This can be accomplished by encouraging patients to use the stairs, walk whenever possible, garden, play actively with children, etc. Examples of moderate physical activity from the Surgeon General's Report on Physical Activity and Health (JAMA 1996;276:522) include:

- Wash and wax a car, or wash windows or floors for 45 minutes
- Garden, dance fast (social), or rake for 30 minutes
- Walk 1¾ miles in 35 minutes (20 min/mile)
- Push a stroller 1½ miles or bicycle 5 miles in 30 minutes
- Stairwalk, shovel snow, or jump rope for 15 minutes

  Exercise should not be exhausting, but it does need to be invigorating and should increase heart rate. Individuals are exercising at the right level of intensity if they can talk without gasping for breath but do not have enough breath to sing (e.g., brisk walking at a pace of 3-4 miles per hour, like walking to catch a bus). For motivated patients able and willing to take their pulse, a reasonable goal is to exercise at 60-80% of maximal heart rate (220 – age [years]). Additionally, exercise does not need to be done all at one time during the day to receive health benefits. The important factor is to accumulate at least 30 minutes of moderate physical activity all or most days of the week (which can be split in three 10-minute blocks). Health benefits may plateau at 3500 kcal per week, the equivalent of moderately intense jogging or bicycling for 1 hour per day.

C. **Evaluation of the Diabetic Patient Prior to Exercise**
   1. **Coronary Heart Disease.** For patients initiating a moderate-to-high intensity exercise program ($\geq$ 55% of predicted maximal heart rate), an exercise stress test should be considered for individuals at increased risk of cardiovascular disease, including:
      - Age > 35 years
      - Age > 25 years with type 2 diabetes > 10 years (or type 1 diabetes > 15 years)
      - Presence of any additional risk factor for coronary disease (e.g., strong family history, hypertension, dyslipidemia, tobacco use)
      - Presence of microvascular disease (proliferative retinopathy or nephropathy, including microalbuminuria)
      - Peripheral arterial disease
      - Autonomic neuropathy (e.g., orthostatic hypotension)

      For patients with known coronary disease, stress testing is recommended prior to initiating an exercise program to determine ischemic threshold, the likelihood for arrhythmias, and LV function at baseline and during exercise.
   2. **Diabetic Retinopathy.** Patients with active proliferative diabetic retinopathy should be instructed to avoid jarring or straining activities due to the increased risk of vitreous hemorrhage and retinal detachment. The degree of diabetic retinopathy can be used to individualize the exercise program (Table 4.7).

Table 4.7. Considerations for Activity Limitation in Diabetic Retinopathy

Level of Retinopathy	Acceptable Activities	Discouraged Activities	Ocular Reevaluation
No DR	Dictated by medical status	Dictated by medical status	12 months
Mild NPDR	Dictated by medical status	Dictated by medical status	6-12 months
Moderate NPDR	Dictated by medical status	Activities that dramatically elevate BP*	4-6 months
Severe NPDR	Dictated by medical status	Activities that substantially increase systolic BP, Valsalva maneuvers, active jarring+	2-4 months (may require laser surgery)
PDR	Low-impact cardiovascular conditioning‡	Strenuous activities, Valsalva maneuvers, pounding or jarring**	1-2 months (may require laser surgery)

BP = blood pressure, DR = diabetic retinopathy, NPDR = nonproliferative diabetic retinopathy, PDR = proliferative diabetic retinopathy
*   Power lifting, heavy Valsalva
+   Boxing, heavy competitive sports
‡   Swimming, walking, low-impact aerobics, stationary cycling, endurance exercises
**   Weightlifting, jogging, high-impact aerobics, racquet sports, strenuous trumpet playing
From: The American Diabetes Association. Diabetes Care 2003;26(suppl 1).

3. **Other Considerations.** Patients with significant peripheral neuropathy should limit weight bearing and repetitive exercises on feet due the increased risk of foot trauma/ulceration. Recommended physical activities for diabetic patients with loss of protective sensation include swimming, bicycling, light weight lifting, arm/chair exercises, and other non-weight-bearing exercises. Activities that should be avoided include jogging and step exercises. Prolonged walking should also be avoided. Following exercise, feet should be routinely inspected for cuts, bruises or other trauma, and appropriate foot care measures initiated (Chapter 6). For diabetic patients with

autonomic neuropathy (e.g., orthostatic hypotension), adequate hydration and avoidance of exercise in extremes of temperature are particularly important measures.

D. Preparing for Exercise. Well-fitting athletic shoes and polyester or polyester-cotton socks will minimize foot trauma and help keep feet dry. Prior to initiating a new exercise program, individuals with diabetes should be instructed to:

- Check blood glucose levels before and after exercising
- Carry some sort of fasting-acting sugar (e.g., glucose tablets) to treat hypoglycemic episodes
- Drink extra sugar-free liquids before, during, and after exercise
- Wear a diabetes information bracelet or necklace
- Carry a mobile phone or enough change to make a phone call in case of an emergency
- Stop exercising and notify physician if pain develops in legs or chest
- Inspect feet for cuts, blisters, callouses before and after exercise

---

Weight Control

A. Overview. An estimated 1.1 billion adults worldwide are overweight or obese (Lancet 2005;366:1197-209), including 65% of U.S. adults (130 million) (JAMA 2002;288:1723-7), a number that has tripled over the last 2 decades. Obesity increases the risk of all-cause mortality and increases morbidity from type 2 diabetes, hypertension, dyslipidemia, CHD, stroke, gallbladder disease, osteoarthritis, sleep apnea, respiratory disease, and cancer (endometrial, breast, prostate, colon). Obesity is a powerful predictor of who will develop diabetes. Compared to women with a BMI < 25 kg/m^2, women with BMIs of 30-35 kg/m^2 and > 35 kg/m^2 have a 20-fold and 39-fold increased risk of new diabetes, respectively (N Engl J Med 2001;345:7907). Overweight adults are also more likely to have overweight children, contributing to the alarming increase of type 2 diabetes among children and young adults. Weight control improves blood pressure, triglycerides, LDL/HDL cholesterol, blood glucose, and hemoglobin A$_{1c}$, and it can prevent/reverse type 2 diabetes. The American Heart Association has issued scientific statements on obesity and its effects on cardiovascular disease (Circulation 2004;110:2952-67; Circulation 2006;113:898-918).

B. **Evaluation of Overweight/Obesity** (Obesity Res 1998;6:51S-209S; Executive Summary, Arch Intern Med 1998;158:1855-67). All diabetic patients should be stratified by body mass index (BMI) to assess overweight/obesity and by waist circumference to assess abdominal fat content (Table 4.8). Increased waist circumference identifies increased risk for CHD independent of BMI and is a criterion for the metabolic syndrome (Chapter 2). (A desirable waist circumference is height in inches divided by 2.) Patient medications should be reviewed to see if adjustments or substitutions can be made for drugs associated with weight gain, including antidepressants, glucocorticoids, phenothiazines, lithium, cyproheptadine, sulfonylureas, and insulin. It is also important to examine the patient for features suggestive of Cushing's syndrome (truncal obesity, moon facies, ecchymosis, muscle atrophy, edema, striae, acne, hirsutism, osteoporosis, glucose intolerance, hypokalemia) or hypothyroidism (weakness, fatigue, cold intolerance, constipation, dry skin, bradycardia, hyporeflexia). Patients with suspected sleep apnea (cessation of breathing during sleep, snoring, restless sleep, excessive daytime sleepiness ± headaches, memory impairment) should be referred to a specialist.

C. **Treatment of Overweight/Obesity.** The treatment of overweight/obesity requires a combination of dietary restriction, increased physical activity, and behavior modification; patients requiring additional measures may benefit from drug therapy and weight loss surgery (refractory cases). Total caloric intake and energy expenditure (physical activity) should be adjusted to achieve and maintain a desirable body weight (BMI 21-25 kg/m^2) and waist circumference (< 102 cm in men, < 88 cm in women). A reasonable initial goal is to reduce body weight by 10% over 6 months, which typically requires calorie deficits of 300-500 kcal/d in patients with BMIs of 27-35 kg/m^2 (0.5-1 lb/week) and 500-1000 kcal/d (1-2 lb/week) in patients with BMIs ≥ 35 kg/m^2. Further weight loss can be considered once this goal is achieved. As little as 5% loss in body weight will preferentially decrease peritoneal fat and disproportionately reduce insulin resistance and improve glycemic control. Calorie deficits are best accomplished through a combination of dietary restriction and increased physical activity. It is essential to communicate encouragement, support, and understanding in order to optimize compliance. Other useful behavior modification techniques include self-monitoring, stress management, problem solving (coping with urges and cravings), contingency management (rewarding achieved goals), cognitive restructuring (changing unrealistic goals and improving self-image), and social support (positive reinforcement). Pharmacotherapy (sibutramine, orlistat) can be a useful adjunct but is unlikely to be effective long term without lifestyle modifications. Drug therapy is especially useful for patients with BMIs $\geq$ 30 kg/m^2 or $\geq$ 27 kg/m^2 in the presence of other risk factors (hypertension, dyslipidemia, type 2 diabetes, CHD, sleep apnea).

Rimonabant, a cannaboid receptor 1 (CB1) antagonist marketed in Europe, has shown efficacy as a treatment for obesity. In RIO-Diabetes, 1047 obese or overweight patients with type 2 diabetes were randomized to the same 3 treatments. For the primary endpoint, body weight decreased by 12 lb from baseline with rimonabant 20 mg; significant improvements were also observed for waist circumference (–5.2 cm), HbA$_{1C}$ (–0.6%), HDL cholesterol (+15%), and triglycerides (–9%). The HbA$_{1C}$ target of < 7% recommended by the American Diabetes Association was achieved at 1 year by 53% of patients on rimonabant 20 mg, compared with 27% of patients on placebo (Lancet 2006;368:1660-72). In the Study Evaluating Rimonabant Efficacy in Drug-Naive Diabetic Patients (SERENADE), 262 type 2 diabetic patients were randomized to rimonabant 20 mg/d or placebo. At 6 months, rimonabant resulted in significant lowering of HbA$_{1c}$ from baseline (0.8% vs. 0.3% for placebo, p = 0.002). In addition, rimonabant resulted in significant weight loss (–15 lbs vs. –6 lbs for placebo, p < 0.0001), reduction in waist circumference (p < 0.0001), increased HDL-C (p < 0.0001), and lowering of triglycerides (p = 0.003) (International Diabetes Federation 19th World Diabetes Congress, December 2-6, 2006, Cape Town, South Africa). However, due to concerns over neurological and psychiatric side effects — seizures, depression, anxiety, insomnia, suicidal ideation — the U.S. Food and Drug Administration denied approval of rimonabant pending further investigation into the drug's safety. Physicians prescribing rimonabant should be alert for neurological and psychiatric adverse effects in their patients.

Gastrointestinal surgery (gastric restriction or bypass) should be reserved for motivated patients with extreme obesity (BMI $\geq$ 40 kg/m^2 or $\geq$ 35 kg/m^2 with comorbid conditions) despite nonsurgical intervention. Compared to conventional therapy, bariatric surgery for severe obesity resulted in more weight loss (1.6% increase vs. 16.1% decrease, p < 0.001); higher 2-year and 10-year recovery rates from diabetes, hypertriglyceridemia, low HDL cholesterol, hypertension and hyperuricemia; and lower 2- and 10-year incident rates of diabetes, hypertriglyceridemia, and hyperuricemia (N Engl J Med 2004;351:2683-93). Life-long medical monitoring and nutritional supplementation with minerals and vitamins (especially iron and vitamin D) are required following bariatric surgery.

Table 4.8. Classification of Overweight and Obesity

Category	BMI*	Waist Circumference†	Risk for Type 2 Diabetes, Hypertension, CHD
Underweight	< 18.5	N	N
Normal	18.5 - 24.9	N or ↑	N or ↑
Overweight	25.0 - 29.9	N ↑	Increased High
Obesity, class			
I	30.0 - 34.9	N ↑	High Very high
II	35.0 - 39.9	N or ↑	Very high
III	≥ 40.0	N or ↑	Extremely high

BMI = body mass index, CHD = coronary heart disease, N = not elevated

* Body mass index = weight in kilograms divided by height in meters squared (kg/m^2). Estimated BMI using nonmetric measurements = (weight in pounds x 703) divided by height in inches squared

† Increased waist circumference: men > 102 cm (> 40 inches); women > 88 cm (> 35 inches). Increased waist circumference can be a marker for increased risk even if weight is normal

Adapted from: NHLBI Guideline Report (Obesity Res 1998;6:51S-209S)

Smoking Cessation

Tobacco use increases the risk of micro- and macrovascular complication of diabetes and is one of the most preventable causes of death worldwide. Each year, 430,000 deaths are attributable to tobacco use in the U.S. alone, more than alcohol abuse, automobile accidents, AIDS, homicide, suicide, heroin, and cocaine combined. Compared to age-matched nonsmokers, persons who smoke 1 pack of cigarettes per day are 14 times more likely to die from cancer of the lung, throat or mouth; 4 times more likely to die from cancer of the esophagus; twice as likely to suffer an MI or stroke; and twice as likely to die from heart disease or cancer of the bladder. At any age, the risk of death is doubled in smokers compared with nonsmoking age-matched controls, and the risk associated with smoking is dose dependent. Despite these statistics, many physicians do not routinely ask patients about cigarette smoking or offer counseling about smoking cessation. The increased cardiovascular risk attributable to smoking returns to baseline soon after cessation of tobacco use, emphasizing the importance of intervention. By 12-18 months, most of the increased cardiovascular risk has disappeared, and by 3-5 years, the risk of vascular events is no different than that of a nonsmoker. As a physician, there is virtually nothing more effective at improving a patient's long-term prognosis than convincing and helping him or her to stop smoking. If a physician discusses this topic even briefly with the smoker and makes a strong statement about the medical necessity of discontinuing this habit, a person's chances of permanent cessation of smoking is doubled. The use of bupropion hydrochloride (Zyban) and nicotine replacement therapy (NRT) also increases the chances of successful smoking cessation. Varenicline (Chantix), a new oral nicotine-receptor blocker (also a partial agonist) appears to be the most effective drug therapy for smoking cessation: In a database review of 6 large trials, the likelihood of smoking cessation was 3-fold greater with varenicline than with placebo or bupropion (Cochrane Database Syst Rev 2007;1:CD006103). Rare episodes of suicidal ideation have been reported in persons using varenicline. The use of a nicotine vaccine for smoking cessation is currently under investigation. Recommendations from the U.S. Public Health Service recommendations from Clinical Practice Guidelines for Treating Tobacco Use and Dependence (JAMA 2000;283:3244) are summarized in Table 4.8.

Table 4.9. Strategies to Assist Patients Willing to Quit Smoking

Step	Strategies for Implementation
Help the patient with a quit plan	• Have patient set a quit date, ideally within 2 weeks. • Have patient tell family, friends, and coworkers about quitting and request their understanding and support. • Help patient anticipate withdrawal symptoms and discuss ways to resist urges and cravings (clean the house; take a 5-minute walk; do stretching exercises; put a toothpick, cinnamon gum, or lemon drop in mouth; take several slow deep breaths; brush teeth; call a nonsmoking friend and talk). • Have patient remove tobacco products from their environment: throw out ashtrays; clean clothes, car, carpets. • Encourage patients to learn as much about how to quit smoking as possible. Useful sources for reading materials include: – American Heart Association, 7272 Greenville Avenue, Dallas, TX 75231, (800) 242-8721; www.americanheart.org – American Cancer Society, 1599 Clifton Road, NE, Atlanta, GA 30329, (800) 227-2345; www.cancer.org – National Cancer Institute, Bethesda, MD 20894, (202) 4-CANCER (422-6237); www.nci.nih.gov – *For pregnant women:* American College of Obstetricians and Gynecologists, 409 12th Street, SW, Washington, DC 20024, (202) 638-5577; www.acog.org
Provide practical counseling	• Total abstinence is essential. "Not even a single puff after you quit." • Identify what helped and hindered previous quit attempts. • Discuss challenges/triggers and how to overcome them. • Since alcohol can cause relapse, the patient should consider limiting/abstaining from alcohol while quitting. • Patients should encourage housemates to quit with them or not to smoke in their presence. • Provide a supportive clinical environment while encouraging the patient to quit: "My staff and I are available for you."

Table 4.9. Strategies to Assist Patients Willing to Quit Smoking (cont'd)

Step	Strategies for Implementation
Recommend approved drug therapy	• Recommend the use of first-line drug therapy (Table 6.4) to all smokers trying to quit, except in special circumstances (e.g., medical contraindications, those smoking fewer than 10 cigarettes/day, pregnant/breastfeeding women, adolescent smokers). If drug therapy is used with lighter smokers (10-15 cigarettes/day), consider reducing the dose of NRT; no dosage adjustment is necessary for sustained-release bupropion hydrochloride or varenicline. • Some studies suggest that: (1) varenicline may be more effective than bupropion; (2) bupropion may be more effective than NRT for achieving permanent cessation of tobacco use; and (3) some synergism between bupropion and NRT may exist. There are insufficient data to rank-order these medications, so initial therapy must be guided by factors such as clinician familiarity with the medications, contraindications for selected patients, patient preference, previous patient experience with a specific therapy (positive or negative), and patient characteristics (e.g., history of depression, concerns about weight gain). Sustained-release bupropion hydrochloride and NRT, in particular nicotine gum, have been shown to delay but not prevent weight gain. Sustained-release bupropion hydrochloride and nortriptyline hydrochloride are particularly well suited for patients with a history of depression. • Combining the nicotine patch with either nicotine gum or nicotine nasal spray may increase long-term abstinence rates over those produced by a single form of NRT, based on a meta-analysis. • The nicotine patch is safe in cardiovascular disease. However, the safety of NRT products has not been established for the immediate post-MI period or in unstable angina. • Long-term therapy may be helpful for smokers who report persistent withdrawal symptoms. A minority of individuals who successfully quit smoking use NRT medications (gum, nasal spray, inhaler) long term. The long-term use of these medications does not present a known health risk, and the FDA has approved the use of sustained-release bupropion hydrochloride for long-term maintenance. • Clonidine and nortriptyline (Table 6.4) may be considered when first-line medications are contraindicated or not helpful

Adapted from: The U.S. Public Health Service Clinical Practice Guidelines for Treating Tobacco Use and Dependence (JAMA 2000;283:3244-54). Varenicline was approved for smoking cessation after publication of the original guidelines.

Psychosocial Risk Factor Reduction

Adverse lifestyle behaviors (e.g., smoking, poor diet, sedentary lifestyle), emotional factors (e.g., depression, chronic anger and anxiety), and chronic stressors (e.g., low emotional/social support, low socioeconomic status, work/marital stress, caregiving strain) increase the risk atherosclerosis progression and adverse cardiovascular events (J Am Coll Cardiol 2005;45:637-51; Lancet 2004;364:937-52). These psychosocial factors adversely affect the neurohumoral system, reduce compliance with medical therapy, and increase the risk of cardiovascular events to a similar degree as other major cardiovascular risk factors (Current Atherosclerosis Reports 2006;8:111-118). Increasing evidence indicates that multifactorial prevention efforts including behavioral/psychosocial intervention may effectively treat psychosocial distress and improve outcomes in patients with cardiovascular disease (J Am Coll Cardiol 2005; 45:637-51). It is recommended that physicians incorporate into clinical practice screening for psychosocial risk factors (Table 4.10) and use behavioral techniques to reduce psychosocial stress (Table 4.11) and promote compliance with therapy (Table 4.12). Patients with significant psychosocial distress or behavioral maladjustment should be referred to appropriate specialists.

Table 4.10. Questions to Screen for Psychosocial Risk Factors

1. How would you describe your energy level?
2. How have you been sleeping?
3. How has your mood been recently?
4. What kind of pressure have you been under at work or at home?
5. What do you do to unwind after work or at the end of the day? Do you have difficulty unwinding?
6. Who do you turn to for support?
7. Are there any personal issues that we have not covered that you would like to share?

From: J Am Coll Cardiol 2005;45:637-51.

Table 4.11. Interventions for Psychosocial Risk Factors

Type of Intervention	Targeted Condition	Intensity of Intervention
Exercise training	Psychologic distress	<u>Less Intense</u>: Exercise prescription plus general guidelines. <u>More Intense</u>: Supervised exercise
Nutritional counseling	Management of stress by overeating	<u>Less Intense</u>: Provide nutritional advice. <u>More Intense</u>: Supervised dietary instruction, weight management, behavior modification
Relaxation training	General stress and stress caused by specific situations	<u>Less Intense</u>: Advise patient to initiate relaxation training; provide audiotapes, videotapes, instructional scripts. <u>More Intense</u>: Teach muscle relaxation, imagery, autogenic training, relaxation breathing, biofeedback
Stress management	General stress and stress caused by specific situations	<u>Less Intense</u>: Recommend vacations, hobbies, yoga, relaxing music, pets, pleasurable activities. <u>More Intense</u>: Teach behavioral strategies (e.g., problem-solving, self-monitoring, appropriate goal-setting, relapse-prevention techniques)
Social support	Poor structural or functional support	<u>Less Intense</u>: Provide specific social suggestions (e.g., join walking groups, engage in socially altruistic activities). <u>More Intense</u>: Use staff as a support base, enroll patient in support group, facilitate family involvement
Health information	Specific stress situations (e.g., at work or home) or low health literacy	<u>Less Intense</u>: Provide situation-specific information in form of book, articles, pamphlet, audiotapes, videotapes, websites. <u>More Intense</u>: Discuss and answer patient questions regarding materials related to health and treatment recommendations

From: J Am Coll Cardiol 2005;45:637-51.

Table 4.12. Promoting Effective Adherence to Behavioral Suggestions

1. Use clear and effective communication; make recommendations specific and simple.
2. Schedule follow-up visits to check adherence, especially during the early practice phase, as opposed to the later, more ingrained habit phase.
3. Provide a motivating rationale for the patient's treatment regimen.
4. Reinforce oral suggestions with written ones.
5. Begin with "micro" goals for patients who are resistant to behavior change.
6. Help patients establish realistic goals and expectations.
7. Involve patients in tailoring behavioral suggestions rather than dictating change.
8. Suggest activities commensurate with patients' abilities and that provide positive feedback (factors that tend to promote a sense of pleasure).
9. Openly and candidly explore potential patient barriers to adherence (e.g., lack of personal motivation, time, family support, facilities, or knowledge; fears; job, home or other pressures; cultural issues); assist patients with problem-solving and developing strategies (e.g., self-monitoring approaches, written agreements, relapse prevention) at the time of recommendations.
10. Refer patients with poor structural or functional social support to programs or activities that will enhance adherence by providing social support.

From: J Am Coll Cardiol 2005;45:637-51.

Chapter 5

Glycemic Control in Type 2 Diabetes

Intensive Glycemic Control

A. **Rationale.** Glycemic control is fundamental to the management of type 2 diabetes. Prospective randomized clinical trials such as the United Kingdom Prospective Diabetes Study (UKPDS) have shown that intensive treatment regimens that reduced average HbA_{1c} levels to $\leq 7\%$ ($\sim 1\%$ above the upper limits of normal) resulted in sustained reductions in retinopathy, nephropathy, and neuropathy (p. 162). In addition, metformin reduced the risk of macrovascular complications and all-cause mortality in the UKPDS substudy of obese patients with diabetes in spite of only a modest (0.6%) reduction in HbA_{1c} (p. 163). Epidemiological analyses have shown a continuous relationship between glycemic control and complication rates and no lower limit of HbA_{1c} at which further lowering does not further reduce the risk of complications (i.e., lower is better). Based on these data, efforts should be made to reduce HbA_{1c} to the lowest possible level at which frequent or severe hypoglycemic episodes do not occur. HbA_{1c} levels between 6-7% are readily achieved in most persons with type 2 diabetes, especially near the time of diagnosis and when utilizing drugs that do not cause hypoglycemia (metformin, TZDs, alpha-glucosidase inhibitors, DPP-4 inhibitors, incretin mimetics).

B. **Disadvantages.** The major disadvantages of intensive treatment are weight gain, which is largely due to reduced calorie loss through glycosuria, and hypoglycemia. Weight gain can usually be controlled through diet modification, increased physical activity, and the use of metformin, incretin mimetics or amylin analogs, which have been shown to attenuate the weight gain associated with improved glucose control when used as monotherapy or in combination with other agents. The other major risk of tight glucose control is hypoglycemia, which can be reduced by frequent blood glucose monitoring; alteration of the timing, frequency, and content of meals; adjustment of insulin or insulin secretagogue dosage (if used); and change in exercise/activity patterns. The highest annual rate of hypoglycemic episodes in UKPDS was 2.3%, which   occurred in subjects receiving insulin. Implementation of intensive glycemic therapy also requires expanded health care teams; major professional and patient educational efforts, including comprehensive self-management training; and an enhanced partnership between specialists and primary care providers.

C. **Recent Trials of Intensive vs. Standard Glycemic Control.** Epidemiologic studies have shown a relationship between HbA_{1c} and cardiovascular prognosis in type 2 diabetes, although the exact role for aggressive glucose lowering remained unclear. Data from three large randomized trials comparing intensive vs standard glucose lowering have been recently published. The Veterans Affairs Diabetes Trial (VADT) trial showed no difference between intensive and standard glycemic control on cardiovascular prognosis, although a benefit was suggested for intensive therapy in newly diagnosed diabetic patients and in diabetic subjects with less advanced atherosclerotic vascular disease (less calcified coronary atherosclerotic plaque) at baseline. The Action in Diabetes and Vascular Disease: Preterax and Diamicron Modified Release Controlled Evaluation (ADVANCE) again showed no difference between groups on major cardiovascular events; however, intensive therapy was associated with fewer microvascular renal complications. In contrast, The Action to Control Cardiovascular Risk in Diabetes (ACCORD) trial was halted early due increased mortality in the intensive glycemic control group.

1. **The VADT Study**. In this trial, 1791 patients with type 2 diabetes (97% male, average age 60 years) were randomized to intensive or standard glycemic control. At enrollment, more than 40% of participants had suffered prior cardiovascular events, and most were obese with abnormal lipid profiles and hypertension. Mean HbA_{1c} was 9.5% at baseline, and was reduced to 6.9% and 8.4% in the intensive and standard therapy groups, respectively. Most patients received several oral drugs, and 90% of participants in the intensive group and 74% of the standard group took insulin during most of the

trial. Rosiglitazone was used in 72% of the intensive group and 62% of the standard group by year 3 of the trial; metformin was more commonly used in obese patients and glimepiride in nonobese patients. Drug use varied over the course of the trial to maintain the established HbA_{1c} levels. At 7.5 years follow-up, there was no reduction in the primary endpoint of the trial – stroke, myocardial infarction, congestive heart failure, and cardiovascular death – in the group subjected to intensive glycemic control, similar to the findings of ADVANCE and ACCORD (see below). However, VADT suggested that lowering blood glucose to near normal levels may reduce the risk of major adverse cardiovascular events if therapy is initiated relatively soon after diagnosis, particularly in those with less advanced atherosclerosis as assessed by coronary artery calcium screening, and if episodes of severe hypoglycemia can be avoided (presented at the American Diabetes Association Scientific Sessions, San Francisco, CA, June, 2008). Although the relationship between tight glycemic control and cardiac outcomes was not significant in VADT, both treatment groups had far fewer adverse cardiovascular events than expected: 263 in the standard treatment group and 231 in the intensive treatment group (predicted total cardiovascular events was from 650 to 700); this decrease was attributed to excellent control of cardiovascular risk factors other than blood glucose. Rosiglitazone use was not associated with increased MI or cardiovascular mortality.

2. **The ADVANCE Study.** In this trial, 11,140 patients (at 215 sites in 20 countries) age 55 years or greater with type 2 diabetes diagnosed after age 30 and cardiovascular disease or at least one cardiovascular risk factor were randomized to intensive (HbA_{1c} of 6.5% or less) vs. standard glucose control ($HbA_{1c} \sim 7.0\%$). Patients in the intensive therapy group (n = 5571) received gliclazide (modified release, 30-120 mg/day) and no other sulfonylureas; other glucose-control agents were prescribed as needed to achieve target HbA_1. Patients randomized to the standard treatment group (n = 5569) received glucose-lowering agents other than gliclazide. Primary endpoints were a composite of major macrovascular events (cardiovascular death, nonfatal MI, or nonfatal stroke) and major microvascular events (new or worsening nephropathy or retinopathy). At 5 years

follow-up, the ADVANCE study attained a mean HbA_{1c} of 6.5% in the intensive glycemic control group vs. 7.3% in the standard treatment group (p < 0.001). This reduction was associated with a 10% relative risk reduction for major macrovascular and microvascular complications (18.1% vs. 20.0%, p = 0.01) and a 14% relative risk reduction for major microvascular events (9.4% vs. 10.9%, p = 0.01), primarily due to a 21% reduction in nephropathy (4.1% vs. 5.2%, p = 0.006). There was no significant difference between groups for major macrovascular events such as MI or stroke (p= 0.32). A 9% decrease in new microalbuminuria (p = 0.02) was also documented in the intensive glycemic control group (N Engl J Med 2008;358:2560-2572).

3. **The ACCORD Study.** In this trial, 10,251 type 2 diabetic patients (mean age 62.2 years, mean HbA_{1c} 8.1%) with established cardiovascular disease or additional cardiovascular risk factors were randomized to intensive (HbA_{1c} < 6.0%) vs. standard glycemic control (HbA_{1c} of 7.0-7.9%). After 3.5 years, the trial was suspended due to significantly more deaths from any cause in the intensive therapy group compared to the standard therapy group (p = 0.04). Additionally, the use of intensive therapy did not significantly reduce the primary outcome of major cardiovascular events (cardiovascular death, nonfatal MI, or nonfatal stroke) (p = 0.16). As in VADT, both treatment groups had far fewer adverse cardiovascular events than expected. Hypoglycemia requiring assistance and weight gain > 10 kg occurred more often in the intensive therapy group (p < 0.001). Rosiglitazone use was not associated with increased MI or cardiovascular mortality (N Engl J Med 2008;358:2545-2559).

D. **Patient Selection.** Considered together, the findings of VADT, ADVANCE and ACCORD suggest that ultra-aggressive regimens for lowering blood glucose and driving HbA_{1c} levels below 6% in type 2 diabetes may not be effective or even safe, especially in those with advanced long-standing diabetes and significant atherosclerotic cardiovascular disease at baseline. Importantly, however, VADT indicated that lowering blood sugar levels to near normal through intensive treatment may reduce the risk of major cardiovascular events for type 2 diabetic patients in whom treatment is initiated relatively soon after diagnosis and if severe episodes of hypoglycemia can be avoided. Additionally, the much lower than expected cardiovascular event rate in all treatment groups in VADT and ACCORD, likely due to high use of statins, ARBs/ACE inhibitors and low-dose aspirin, emphasizes the need for these pharmacologic therapies for optimal management of patients with type 2 diabetes.

Over time, two problems typically occur in patients with type 2 diabetes: (1) deterioration of the pancreatic beta cells' ability to produce insulin, and (2) development of cardiovascular disease (arterial atherosclerosis, left ventricular hypertrophy/dysfunction). Early in the course of type diabetes, aggressive therapy using agents such as metformin, TZDs, DPP-4 inhibitors, and alpha glucosidase inhibitors will allow for tight glucose control without causing hypoglycemia. Using these agents early in diabetes is more likely to improve cardiovascular prognosis, as the toxicity of hyperglycemia is avoided without incurring the liability of hypoglycemic spells. However, as diabetes progresses and the pancreas fails, insulin therapy is required, often in the setting of occult or manifest cardiovascular disease. Aggressive therapy needed to achieve low HbA$_{1c}$ targets of < 6.0% in these patients (i.e., with long-standing diabetes) may increase the risk of cardiovascular mortality and bouts of severe hypoglycemia and is not recommended. Although there are few absolute contraindications to intensive glycemic therapy, aggressive tight control should not be attempted in noncompliant patients or in patients with frequent/severe hypoglycemic episodes. Also, older individuals with long-standing diabetes and occult or manifest coronary atherosclerosis may be vulnerable to increased mortality as well as permanent cerebral injury from prolonged/severe hypoglycemia and may not be good candidates for intensive glycemic control.

General Approach to Intensive Glycemic Control

The American Diabetes Association (ADA) recommends initiating glycemic therapy for persons with preprandial plasma glucose levels > 150 mg/dL, bedtime plasma glucose levels > 180 mg/dL, pre-prandial whole blood glucose levels > 140 mg/dL, or bedtime whole blood glucose levels > 160 mg/dL. Adult nonpregnant patients should receive aggressive enough treatment to obtain HbA_{1c} levels of 7% or below. However, the American Association of Clinical Endocrinologists (AACE)/American College of Endocrinology (ACE), and the International Diabetes Federation all recommend tighter glycemic control (HbA_{1c} < 6.5%; Table 3.2, p. 31). The Canadian Diabetes Association has recommended the goal of therapy to be a normal HbA_{1c} (< 6%) if this can be achieved without unacceptable side effects (hypoglycemia); as of 2006, the ADA has added this as an optional goal for treatment. However, these recommendations were issued prior to the results of VADT, ADVANCE, and ACCORD, which have important implications for patient selection for intensive glycemic control (pp. 64-67).

A. **Therapeutic Lifestyle Changes.** Diet and exercise are the cornerstones for successful management of type 2 diabetes. Caloric restriction, weight loss, and increased physical activity will improve insulin resistance, hyperglycemia, hypertension, and lipid profile. Lifestyle changes also improve the efficacy of other diabetic therapies. In some obese patients, lifestyle changes may appear to reverse diabetes. For most patients, however, once diabetes is diagnosed, at least a relative insulin deficiency is present, and pharmacologic therapy is usually required; lifestyle changes alone almost invariably fail within months. Guidelines for medical nutritional therapy, weight loss, and physical activity are described in Chapter 4.

B. **Pharmacologic Therapy.** Traditional management of hyperglycemia involved starting with a single agent, increasing that agent to the maximum recommended dose, then waiting for HbA_{1c} levels to rise before advancing/changing therapy. This passive approach has proven to be ineffective at controlling diabetes and preventing complications. Multiple classes of oral agents are now available which can be used at lower doses in combination to improve glycemic control, reduce side effects, and address the fundamental defects in type 2 diabetes—insulin resistance, beta-cell secretory defect, increased glucose production by the liver, and decreased incretin production from the intestine. Combination therapy to handle most or all of these defects should be instituted early in the treatment course to achieve/maintain normoglycemia, improve insulin resistance and preserve beta-cell function, rather than initiated as a reaction to uncontrolled, symptomatic hyperglycemia.

Drug Classes Used for Glycemic Control (Tables 5.1, 5.2)

There are five functional classes of oral diabetes agents, which work primarily by: (1) augmenting insulin secretion (secretagogues); (2) decreasing hepatic glucose production (metformin); (3) improving insulin activity in the muscle, liver, and adipocyte (thiazolidinediones [TZDs]); (4) decreasing glucose absorption from the gastrointestinal tract (alpha-glucosidase inhibitors); or (5) increasing incretin levels (incretin mimetics or DPP-4 inhibitors) (Table 5.1). In addition, there are three classes of subcutaneous injectable agents: insulin, incretin mimetics (exenatide), and amylin analogs (pramlintide). This section reviews the various drug classes used for glycemic control in type 2 diabetes.

A. **Insulin Secretagogues: Stimulation of Pancreatic Beta Cells to Produce More Insulin.** Antidiabetic drugs that act by increasing insulin secretion are called secretagogues, and they can be separated into two groups: sulfonylureas and the glitinides. <u>Sulfonylureas</u> are one of the oldest classes of antidiabetic agents, and many are available. The two most common adverse effects associated with sulfonylureas are hypoglycemia and weight gain. Second-generation sulfonylureas (glyburide, glipizide, glimepiride) are more effective at lowering HbA_{1c} than older agents (e.g., chlorpropamide) and are associated with fewer adverse effects. The lowest rate of hypoglycemia and weight gain is with glimepiride. Sulfonylureas, with the exception of glimepiride, abolish ischemic preconditioning of the myocardium in some patients, predisposing to larger infarcts in the setting of coronary occlusion and loss of ST segment elevation so that fibrinolytic therapy is not utilized. The <u>glitinide</u> secretagogues are a newer class and include two currently available products: nateglinide and repaglinide. Both products are approved for use as monotherapy or in combination with metformin. Repaglinide is also approved for use with TZDs. Compared to sulfonylureas, these agents have a shorter half-life (shorter duration of action) and a reduced risk of hypoglycemia. Because of their short half-life, glitinides are administered at meals to improve postprandial glycemic control, which may result in less weight gain and potentially less atherosclerosis and fewer cardiac events than the longer-acting sulfonylureas. In one study, despite similar improvements in HbA_{1c}, nateglinide and repaglinide reduced inflammation and atherosclerosis better than sulfonylureas, probably due to superior reductions in post-prandial glucose levels (Circulation 2004;110:214-219). The secretagogues have traditionally been employed as first-line therapy because for many years they were the only oral agents available to treat hyperglycemia. Their ability to rapidly lower blood glucose levels is valuable in the initial short-term management of hyperglycemia, but the effect is not durable (Figure 5.1) and other agents must be added to maintain normoglycemia in the majority of patients. Traditionally a secretagogue would be increased to the maximal FDA-approved dose before adding other agents to the glycemic regimen. However, data suggest that maximal augmentation of insulin secretion typically occurs using 25-50% of the maximum recommended dose, which has resulted in a trend toward use of a low-dose secretagogue in early combination therapy, and not increasing the secretagogue dose beyond half-maximum. The triple combination of a secretagogue, metformin, and a TZD is now FDA approved.

Table 5.1. Oral Glycemic Agents Used for Type 2 Diabetes

Drug Class	Antidiabetic Agents	Mechanisms of Action
Thiazolidinediones (TZDs)	Rosiglitazone (Avandia) Pioglitazone (Actos)	Increased insulin sensitivity; preservation of beta cell function; decreased hepatic glucose output
Biguanides	Metformin (Glucophage)	Decreased hepatic glucose output; mild increased insulin sensitivity
Alpha-glucosidase inhibitors	Acarbose (Precose) Miglitol (Glyset)	Delayed GI absorption of carbohydrates; increased incretin production

Table 5.1. Oral Glycemic Agents Used for Type 2 Diabetes (cont'd)

Drug Class	Antidiabetic Agents	Mechanisms of Action
Insulin secretagogues *Sulfonylureas*	Chlorpropamide (Diabinese) Glipizide (Glucotrol/XL) Glyburide (DiaBeta, Micronase, Glynase) Glimepiride (Amaryl)	Increased insulin release
Glitinides	Nateglinide (Starlix) Repaglinide (Prandin)	Increased insulin release
Dipeptidyl peptidase-4 (DPP-4) inhibitors	Sitagliptin (Januvia)	Increased GLP-1 levels; augmentation of glucose-stimulated insulin release and suppression of glucagon production; preservation of beta cell function
Combination TZD + biguanide	Rosiglitazone + metformin (Avandamet) Pioglitazone + metformin (Actoplusmet)	Increased insulin sensitivity; decreased hepatic glucose output; preservation of beta cell function
Combination sulfonylurea + biguanide	Glipizide + metformin (Metaglip) Glyburide + metformin (Glucovance)	Increased insulin secretion; decreased hepatic glucose output
Combination TZD + sulfonylurea	Rosiglitazone + glimepiride (Avandaryl) Pioglitazone + glimepiride (Duetact)	Increased insulin secretion; increased insulin sensitivity; preservation of beta cell function

Table 5.2a. Antidiabetic Therapies for Type 2 Diabetes: Diet/Exercise, Sulfonylureas/Glitinides, Metformin[†]

	Diet/Exercise	Sulfonylureas/Glitinides	Metformin
Primary mechanism	Decreased insulin resistance	Increased insulin secretion	Decreased hepatic glucose output
Typical ↓ in HbA_{1c}*	0.5-2.0	1.0-2.0	1.0-2.0
Typical starting dose	Caloric restriction to decrease weight by 1-2 kg/month; increase moderate exercise to ≥ 30 minutes daily	glyburide (1.25 mg/d) glipizide (2.5 mg/d) glimepiride (1-2 mg/d) nateglinide (60 mg)[¶] repaglinide (0.5 mg)[¶]	500 mg bid immediately after breakfast and dinner
Maximal dose	Can use meal substitutes and add orlistat or sibutramine	glyburide (20 mg/d) glipizide (40 mg/d) glimepiride (8 mg/d) nateglinide (120 mg)[¶] repaglinide (4 mg)[¶]	2550 mg/d (850 mg with meals or 1 gm bid plus 500 mg at noon or bedtime)
Common or severe adverse effects	Joint pain	Hypoglycemia, weight gain	GI symptoms (especially diarrhea), lactic acidosis (rare)
Advantages	No medications, improves insulin sensitivity, improves nearly all other CV risk factors	Well established, ↓ microvascular risk, nateglinide/repaglinide target postprandial glycemia and may cause less weight gain, less hypoglycemia, and ↑ risk of cardiovascular events	↓ macrovascular risk, facilitates weight loss, improves lipid profile, no hypoglycemia, ↑ fibrinolysis, ↓ CRP, improves endothelial function
Disadvantages	Poor compliance	Hypoglycemia, weight gain, hyperinsulinemia, multiple daily dosing (nateglinide/repaglinide), lack of CV benefit in outcome trials	Adverse GI effects, many contraindications, lactic acidosis (rare), anemia

Table 5.2a. Antidiabetic Therapies for Type 2 Diabetes: Diet/Exercise, Sulfonylureas/Glitinides, Metformin† (cont'd)

	Diet/Exercise	Sulfonylureas/Glitinides	Metformin
Combination products	—	glyburide/metformin glipizide/metformin rosiglitazone/glimepiride pioglitazone/glimepiride	glyburide/metformin glipizide/metformin rosiglitazone/metformin pioglitazone/metformin sitagliptin/metformin

Also see Tables 5.1-5.4 and Chapter 11 for additional product information
* Drop in HbA_{1c} depends on level at time of initiation of therapy
† In addition to the antidiabetic therapies listed above, pramlintide is an amylin mimetic indicated for patients who used mealtime insulin therapy and have failed to achieve desired glucose control. See p. 180 for pramlintide drug summary.
¶ Administer before meals

Table 5.2b. Antidiabetic Therapies for Type 2 Diabetes: DPP-4 Inhibitors, TZDs, Alpha-Glucosidase Inhibitors†

	DPP-4 Inhibitor	TZDs	Alpha-Glucosidase Inhibitors
Primary mechanism	Increased incretin (GLP-1, GIP) levels	Increased insulin sensitivity	Delayed GI absorption of carbohydrates
Typical ↓ in HbA_{1c}*	0.6-1.0	0.5-1.9	0.5-1.0
Typical starting dose	sitagliptin (100 mg/d)	rosiglitazone (2 mg/d) pioglitazone (15 mg/d)	acarbose (25 mg)‡ miglitol (25 mg)‡
Maximal dose	sitagliptin (200 mg/d)	rosiglitazone (8 mg/d) pioglitazone (45 mg/d)	acarbose (100 mg)‡ miglitol (100 mg)‡
Common or severe adverse effects	Skin lesions, including Stevens-Johnson syndrome; angioedema, anaphylaxis (rare)	Edema, weight gain, macular edema, CHF, anemia, increased risk of long-bone fracture	Flatulence, GI discomfort

**Table 5.2b. Antidiabetic Therapies for Type 2 Diabetes:
DPP-4 Inhibitors, TZDs, Alpha-Glucosidase Inhibitors (cont'd)**[†]

	DPP-4 Inhibitor	TZDs	Alpha-Glucosidase Inhibitors
Advantages	Increases incretin (GLP-1, GIP) levels. Increases insulin release and suppresses glucagon and post-prandial glucose levels. May preserve beta-cell function and decrease hepatic glucose production	No hypoglycemia, glycemic durability, non-glycemic CV risk reduction, ↓ insulin resistance, once-daily dosing, possible beta cell preservation; ↓ in PAI₁, metalloproteinases, blood pressure, and microalbuminuria	Targets postprandial glycemia, rare hypoglycemia, nonsystemic
Disadvantages	—	Weight gain, edema, slow onset of action, potential ↑ risk of CHF, anemia, long-bone fractures, macular edema	More complex (3 times daily) dosing schedule, adverse GI effects, decrease dose in chronic kidney disease
Combination products	sitagliptin/ metformin	rosiglitazone/metformin rosiglitazone/glimepiride pioglitazone/glimepiride pioglitazone/metformin	None

Also see Tables 5.1-5.4 and Chapter 11 for additional product information

*   Drop in HbA$_{1c}$ depends on level at time of initiation of therapy.

†   In addition to the antidiabetic therapies listed above, pramlintide is an amylin mimetic indicated for patients who used mealtime insulin therapy and have failed to achieve desired glucose control. See p. 180 for pramlintide drug summary.

‡   Administer with meals

Table 5.2c. Antidiabetic Therapies for Type 2 Diabetes: Incretin Mimetics, Insulin[†]

	Incretin Mimetic	Insulin[§]
Primary mechanism	Slowed gastric emptying, increased insulin secretion and release, suppressed glucagon production	Increased insulin levels
Typical ↓ in HbA$_{1c}$*	0.4-1.1	1.5-2.5 (dependent on starting HbA$_{1c}$)
Typical starting dose	exenatide 5 mcg bid SC	Depends on insulin regimen, patient characteristics, HbA$_{1c}$
Maximal dose	exenatide 10 mcg bid SC	None
Common/severe adverse effects	Nausea, acute pancreatitis	Hypoglycemia, weight gain
Advantages	Weight loss, beta-cell rejuvenation, decreased glucagon production, decreased post-prandial glucose	Good control with intensive therapy, some but not all can be used in gestational diabetes
Disadvantages	Nausea	Hypoglycemia, multiple daily injections, weight gain
Combination products	None	Humulog Mix 75/25, Humulog Mix 50/50, Humulin Mix 70/30, Humulin Mix, 50/50, Novolog Mix 70/30, Novolin 70/30

Also see Tables 5.1-5.4 and Chapter 11 for additional product information

*   Drop in HbA$_{1c}$ depends on level at time of initiation of therapy.

†   In addition to the antidiabetic therapies listed above, pramlintide is an amylin mimetic indicated for patients who used mealtime insulin therapy and have failed to achieve desired glucose control. See p. 180 for pramlintide drug summary.

§   Also see pp. 187-188

B. **Metformin: Reduction of Glucose Output by the Liver.** The primary action of metformin, the only biguanide available in the U.S., is to reduce production of glucose by the liver and kidney. Among 753 obese diabetic subjects randomized to metformin or conventional care (diet) in UKPDS, metformin reduced the risk of diabetes-related complications by 32% (p = 0.002) and diabetes-related death by 42% (p = 0.017) at 10.7 years despite only a 0.6% lowering of the HbA_{1c}. In addition, the rate of elevation of the HbA_{1c} over time was less with metformin than it was with a sulfonylurea (Lancet 1998;352:854-6). Metformin also reduced the progression from IGT to diabetes by 31% at 2.8 years in the Diabetes Prevention Program, with a greater decrease in younger subjects (N Engl J Med 2002;346:393-403). Because the mode of action does not increase pancreatic insulin secretion, hypoglycemic episodes usually do not occur. Metformin also has an anorexic effect, helping to curb the weight gain associated with improved glycemic control. Given these effects, metformin has been recommended by both the ADA and the EASD as initial monotherapy for most type 2 diabetic patients, and is desirable to include as a component of combination therapy. Metformin is usually initiated at a starting dose of 500 mg twice daily after meals and increased at two weekly intervals to a target dose of 1000 mg twice daily. Alternatively, it is reasonable to titrate metformin to 500 mg twice daily and then add a low dose of a thiazolidinedione and/or secretagogue before increasing the dose of metformin. The most common adverse events include abdominal pain, nausea, and diarrhea, especially if taken on an empty stomach. These side effects can be minimized by starting metformin at a low dose at the end of a meal and increasing the dose on a biweekly basis and/or using the extended-release formulation. Bicarbonate therapy is no longer recommended. Lactic acidosis is a rare but serious complication of metformin therapy, particularly in individuals with renal, hepatic, or cardiac dysfunction or advancing age. Early manifestations may be subtle (malaise), but abdominal pain, obtundation, hypotension, and tachypnea quickly ensue. Lactic acid levels usually exceed 5 mcg/mL. Lactic acidosis requires emergent and prolonged hemodialysis until lactic acid levels return to normal. Lactic acidosis is not a dose-related phenomenon, so there is no dose of metformin that can safely be administered to patients with an elevated serum creatinine. Contraindications to metformin use are listed in Table 5.3. Creatinine

Table 5.3. Contraindications to Metformin Use

- Age $\geq$ 80 years with decreased creatinine clearance
- Renal disease or renal dysfunction (serum creatinine $\geq$ 1.5 mg/dL in males or $\geq$ 1.4 mg/dL in females or abnormal creatinine clearance [< 50-70 mL/min]).
- Acute or chronic systolic dysfunction leading to tissue underperfusion and metabolic acidosis
- Known hypersensitivity to metformin
- Clinical or laboratory evidence of liver disease
- Acute or chronic metabolic acidosis, including DKA, with or without coma
- Metformin should be temporarily discontinued for surgical procedures and at time of or prior to radiologic studies involving IV administration of iodinated contrast materials and for 48 hours after procedure (until renal function can be documented as being normal).
- Metformin should be promptly withheld in the presence of any condition associated with hypoxemia, dehydration, or sepsis

clearance (CrCl) should be monitored in patients receiving metformin, because at least 15% of diabetic patients will have an abnormal CrCl despite a normal serum creatinine and no microalbuminuria. Metformin should not be started in patients $\geq$ 80 years unless CrCl is normal, and should not be started or continued in patients with CrCl < 50 mL/min. For a CrCl of 50-70 mL/ min, metformin could be maintained at a lower dose in the setting of stable renal function but should be discontinued if renal function is deteriorating. Chronic use may result in anemia due to malabsorption of vitamin B_{12}.

C. **Thiazolidinediones (TZDs): Stimulation of Glucose Uptake by Muscle and Adipose Tissues.** TZDs bind to the peroxisome proliferator-activated receptor-gamma (PPAR-gamma) receptor and are unique in their ability to alter the expression of genes that modulate insulin action and lipid metabolism. TZDs decrease insulin resistance by improving insulin sensitivity in muscle, liver, and adipose tissue. They also improve surrogate markers of beta cell function and restore first-phase insulin release (the earliest beta cell change in type 2 diabetes), suggesting an important rejuvenating effect on the pancreatic beta cell, which normally deteriorates in function over time (Figure 2.4, p. 20). The net effect of

TZDs is to decrease circulating hyperinsulinemia while improving glycemic control. Both rosiglitazone and pioglitazone have been shown to slow atherosclerosis as measured by carotid intimal thickness using carotid ultrasound (STARR study: presented at the American College of Cardiology meeting, March, 2007, New Orleans, LA, also available at theheart.org; CHICAGO study: JAMA 2006;296:2572-2581). The PERISCOPE study recently reported that pioglitazone halted coronary plaque growth, whereas glimepiride did not (JAMA 2008;299:1561-1573). The VICTORY study showed a trend toward less progression of atherosclerosis in saphenous vein bypass grafts post-CABG in patients with diabetes treated with rosiglitazone compared to placebo (presented at the American College of Cardiology meeting, March, 2008, Chicago, IL; also available at theheart.org). .

Hypoglycemia with TZD monotherapy is rare and not severe. More frequent and severe hypoglycemia may occur when TZDs are used in combination with secretagogues or insulin but not with metformin. Preservation of beta-cell function and improvement in insulin sensitivity are the major rationales for use of TZDs early in the course of type 2 diabetes. These agents also exert numerous effects on the vasculature and lipid metabolism that may be particularly beneficial in patients with type 2 diabetes (Table 5.4). Rosiglitazone and pioglitazone are the only TZDs currently available in the U.S. Both agents are indicated as monotherapy in patients with type 2 diabetes, or as combination therapy with a sulfonylurea, metformin, exenatide, or DPP-4 inhibitor. Rosiglitazone is not recommended for use with insulin or nitrates. If pioglitazone is coadministered with insulin, only a low dose (15 mg/d) should be used. TZDs lead to more sustained glycemic control than is seen with sulfonylureas or metformin, perhaps due to their beta cell effect. In A Diabetes Outcome Progression Trial (ADOPT), 4360 treatment-naive patients with type 2 diabetes were randomized to 4 years of treatment with rosiglitazone, metformin, or glyburide. The primary outcome was time to monotherapy failure (FPG > 180 mg/dL). The cumulative incidence of monotherapy failure at 5 years was significantly less for rosiglitazone (15%) compared to either metformin (21%) or glyburide (34%), representing risk reductions of 32% and 63%, respectively (p < 0.001 for both comparisons) (Figure 5.1) (N Engl J Med 2006;355:2427-43). TZDs may cause weight gain and edema when administered at high doses due to increased sodium absorption in the very distal renal tubule; combination use with insulin or a secretagogue appears to further increase the incidence of fluid accumulation, since insulin is also a salt-retaining hormone. In rare instances, due to an increase in plasma volume of as much as 6%, progression to macular edema or heart failure may occur if the drug is not stopped. In ADOPT, congestive heart failure was seen more often in the rosiglitazone (1.9%) and metformin (1.8%) groups than in the sulfonylurea group (0.6%). Peripheral edema usually resolves within 3-14 days of discontinuing the TZD. Weight gain and edema can be minimized by initiating therapy with low doses (rosiglitazone 2 mg, pioglitazone 15 mg) followed by slow upward titration at 3-6 month intervals. Since TZDs act on the distal tubule of the kidney to retain salt and water, spironolactone and amiloride, but not loop diuretics or thiazides, may be useful to prevent/minimize the edema. However, if spironolactone or eplerenone therapy is initiated, serum potassium levels should be checked at days 3, 10, and 21. High-dose ACE inhibitors, ARBs, and fibrates may also be useful to prevent TZD-induced edema. In contrast, concomitant treatment with dihydropyridine calcium antagonists and NSAIDs may worsen the edema. TZDs have not been studied in patients with New York Heart Association Class 3 or 4 cardiac status and at this time are not approved for use in these patients. TZDs do not have an adverse effect on myocardial structure or function but do increase plasma volume. TZDs are also associated with a modest drop in the hematocrit, either due to hemodilution or a decrease in bone marrow production of erythrocytes. A post-hoc analysis of reported adverse events in ADOPT showed that rosiglitazone was associated with an increased rate of long-bone but not hip or vertebral fractures. Subsequently, pioglitazone was shown to have the same effect, as well as an increased prevalence of osteoporosis, due to decreased numbers or activity of osteoblasts. The combination of fibrates and TZDs has been shown in rare case reports to be associated with a dramatic lowering of HDL cholesterol, which resolves on stopping therapy. Troglitazone, an older TZD, was removed from the market because of idiosyncratic hepatotoxicity. Hepatic failure is not a class effect with these agents; neither rosiglitazone nor pioglitazone have been associated with liver dysfunction, and routine monitoring of liver enzymes is not necessary when TZDs are administered.

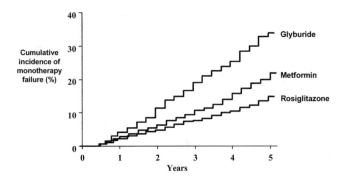

Figure 5.1. Results of ADOPT

In the ADOPT trial, 4360 recently diagnosed type 2 diabetic patients were randomized to 4 years of treatment with rosiglitazone, metformin, or glyburide. Rosiglitazone monotherapy had the most durable effect on glycemic control, reducing the risk of treatment failure (FPG > 180 mg/dL), the primary outcome of the study, by 32% compared to metformin (15% vs. 21%, p < 0.001) and by 63% compared to glyburide (15% vs. 34%, p < 0.001) (N Engl J Med 2006;355:2427-43).

D. **Alpha-Glucosidase Inhibitors: Reduction of Glucose Absorption by the Gut.** Acarbose and miglitol are alpha-glucosidase inhibitors that act by delaying carbohydrate absorption in the small intestine. Among patients with IGT, acarbose reduced the risk of new diabetes by 25%, new hypertension by 34%, and cardiovascular events by 49% in STOP-NIDDM (Lancet 2002;359:2072-77). Cardiac events were also reduced in studies of type 2 diabetes (JAMA 2003;290:468-94), and acarbose was shown to reduce carotid intimal-medial thickening, a marker for early atherosclerosis, by 50% (Stroke 2004;35:1073-8). Reductions in atherosclerosis and cardiovascular events are thought to be due to lowering of postprandial glucose, free fatty acids, and triglycerides.

Table 5.4. Metabolic and Other Effects of Oral Diabetic Agents

	TZDs	Metformin	Sulfonylureas/ Glitinides	Acarbose
Small dense LDL	↓	NC	Unknown	Unknown
LDL cholesterol	↑	↓ or NC	NC	NC
HDL cholesterol	↑ ↑	↑ or NC	NC	NC
Triglycerides	↓ or NC	↓	NC	↓
Free fatty acids‡	↓ ↓ ↓	↓ ↓	↓	↓
Insulin sensitivity	Improved	Improved or NC	NC	NC
Blood pressure	↓	NC	NC	↓
Endothelial function	Improved	0	Unknown	Unknown
PAI-1*	↓ ↓	↓ or NC	NC	NC
C-reactive protein†	↓ ↓	↓	NC	NC
Rate of decline of beta cell function	Improved	NC	Accelerated (ADOPT)	NC
Delay/prevent diabetes	Yes	Yes	No	Yes
Cardiovascular outcomes	Possibly improved with pioglitazone (PROACTIVE); uncertain with rosiglitazone	Improved (UKPDS 34)	No effect (or possibly increased events)	Possibly improved (STOP-NIDDM)
Adverse effects	Mild dilutional anemia, weight gain, edema, CHF, macular edema, long-bone fracture	GI effects (mainly diarrhea), lactic acidosis (rare)	Hypoglycemia, weight gain	Flatulence, diarrhea, liver disease in patients with renal decompensation

Glitinides = nateglinide, repaglinide; sulfonylureas = chlorpropamide, glipizide, glyburide, glimepiride; TZDs = thiazolidinediones (rosiglitazone, pioglitazone)
* Lower levels of PAI-1 are associated with enhanced fibrinolytic capacity
† Lower levels of CRP indicate less systemic inflammation; elevated levels are associated with increased cardiac risk
‡ Free fatty acids worsen insulin sensitivity and are toxic to pancreatic beta cells
↓ = decreased, ↑ = increased, NC = no change

Alpha-glucosidase inhibitors are approved for use as monotherapy or combination therapy and are administered at the beginning of each main meal. The main advantage of these agents is that they are only minimally absorbed from the GI tract and are not associated with hypoglycemia or weight gain. However, they are less effective at lowering HbA_{1c} levels than other oral agents and frequently cause flatulence, which substantially reduces long-term compliance. Alpha-glucosidase inhibitors are best tolerated in patients without diarrhea or symptoms of irritable bowel syndrome at baseline. Compliance may be facilitated by initiating therapy with a half-tablet of the lowest dose followed by slow upward titration at half-tablet increments. Additionally, by limiting ingestion of starches and sucrose, flatulence can be markedly reduced, but efficacy is greatest in those who consume a high-carbohydrate diet. Efficacy can be monitored by observing a decrease in postprandial glucose excursions. Alpha-glucosidase inhibitors are contraindicated in patients with certain diseases of the gastrointestinal tract (e.g., inflammatory bowel disease, irritable bowel syndrome, malabsorption) and should only be used in low doses in chronic renal disease and avoided if CrCl < 25 mL/min because it has not been studied in populations with low creatinine clearance, and the small amount absorbed is excreted renally.

E. **Dipeptidyl Peptidase-4 (DPP-4) Inhibitors.** Glucagon-like peptide-1 (GLP-1) and glucose-dependent insulinotropic polypeptide (GIP) are glucoregulatory *incretin hormones* released from endocrine cells in the mucosa of the small intestine in response to food. GLP-1 and GIP bind to receptors on the pancreatic alpha and beta cells, where they stimulate insulin release, suppress glucagon secretion, and reduce postprandial glucose and lipid levels. Furthermore, at least in animal studies, GLP-1 has been shown to improve pancreatic alpha and beta cell mass by increasing proliferation and decreasing apoptosis of these cells.

The incretin system is impaired in type 2 diabetes, and the decline in production in GLP-1 coincides with onset of the disease. To prevent the breakdown of GLP-1 and GIP by the enzyme DPP-4 and prolong GLP-1 and GIP's effects, an oral DPP-4 inhibitor, sitagliptin, has been approved for use in the U.S.

Like the incretin mimetics (see below), DPP-4 inhibitors stimulate insulin release, suppress glucagon secretion, and reduce postprandial glucose, free fatty acid, and triglyceride levels. Unlike incretin mimetics, DPP-4 inhibitors do not delay gastric emptying or result in weight loss or nausea. Early studies suggest that DPP-4 inhibitors may improve beta cell function.

DPP-4 inhibitors are approved for use as monotherapy or in combination with sulfonylureas, TZDs, or metformin. Their use with insulin has not yet been studied or approved.

F. **Incretin Mimetics.** Incretins are a series of glucoregulatory hormones secreted in direct proportion to meal size – even before blood glucose levels rise – from specialized endocrine cells in the gut. Incretins bind to receptors on pancreatic beta cells, stimulating the release of insulin and reducing the release of glucagon. The defining feature of an incretin is that it results in glucose-dependent insulin secretion. Production of glucoregulatory incretins is decreased at the onset of type 2 diabetes. Since the most important incretin, GLP-1, is quickly broken down by DPP-4 when injected subcutaneously, methods to replace GLP-1 activity have been developed. Exenatide, an incretin mimetic originally isolated from the Gila monster, mimics the effects of GLP-1 on its receptor and is not broken down by DPP-4.

Exenatide lowers post-prandial glucose levels by increasing insulin release and by decreasing glucagon release and gastric emptying in response to a meal. Variable weight loss also occurs, possibly due to delayed gastric emptying, induced satiety through a direct effect on GLP-1 receptors in the hypothalamus or nausea, which is a recognized side effect in approximately 50% of patients. Potentially, exenatide may increase beta-cell mass by stimulating proliferation and suppressing apoptosis of these cells. To date, this has only been shown with high GLP-1 levels in animal studies; in humans, high GLP-1 levels following gastric bypass surgery have been associated with hyperinsulinemia, hypoglycemia, and at least one case of an insulinoma. In human studies, the pro-insulin to insulin ratio is decreased with exenatide, indicating improved beta-cell function.

Exenatide must be administered by subcutaneous injection twice daily. An acylated GLP-1 derivative (liraglutide), which is bound to albumin to protect it from DPP-4 degradation, is under development and can be administered once daily with similar effects to those of exenatide. In addition, long-acting (administered once weekly) exenatide is being developed.

Exenatide is approved for use as add-on therapy with metformin, sulfonylureas, metformin + sulfonylureas, or TZDs. Initiating low-dose therapy once or twice daily reduces the incidence and severity of nausea, allowing most patients to advance to and tolerate the 10-mcg dose.

G. **Amylin Analogs.** Amylin is a neurohormone co-secreted with insulin from the pancreatic beta cells in response to eating. Amylin slows gastric emptying, which can result in early satiety, decreased food intake, and weight loss. It also suppresses glucagon release in the postprandial state which, in conjunction with decreased gastric emptying, results in lower postprandial glucose levels. Amylin also suppresses hepatic glucose production. Pramlintide (Symlin), an amylin-mimetic administered by subcutaneous injection before eating, has been approved for use in type 1 diabetes and in type 2 diabetic subjects who require insulin to lower postprandial glucose levels and body weight. Common side effects include hypoglycemia, nausea, vomiting, and abdominal pain. The necessity for injections before each meal has limited the utilization of pramlintide therapy.

H. **Insulins.** Insulins can be classified according to their mode of action.
   1. **Fast-acting insulins.** These analogues have a rapid onset of action and a short duration of activity so that physiological insulin levels can be achieved postprandially without untoward risk of postprandial hypoglycemia. Fast-acting insulins include lispro (Humalog), aspart (Novolog), and glulisine (Apidra). These insulins have an onset of action at 5-15 minutes, peak activity at 30-90 minutes, and a duration of action up to 5 hours.
   2. **Short-acting insulin.** Regular insulin is the only available short-acting insulin. Its use as a subcutaneous insulin has become outmoded and should now be confined to intravenous therapy. Due to its late peak and longevity of action, postprandial hyperglycemia/

hypoglycemia may occur following subcutaneous administration. Regular insulins have an onset of action at 30-60 minutes, peak activity at 2-3 hours, and a duration of action up to 6 hours.

3. **Intermediate-acting insulin.** The only intermediate-acting insulin that is now available in the United States is NPH. The major disadvantage of NPH is that it is a suspension and not a solution so that multiple inversions of the vial or pen are needed—but seldom performed—before injection. As a result of this and other variables (e.g., dose and site of injection), the absorption of subcutaneous NPH is erratic, resulting in unpredictable periods of hyperglycemia and hypoglycemia. Because of this, lower doses of NPH must be utilized and targets for glycemic control are not reached. NPH is often administered once daily at bedtime in combination with oral agents or twice daily when utilized as a basal insulin in both type 1 and type 2 diabetes. NPH has an onset of action at 2-4 hours, peak activity at 4-10 hours, and duration of action of 10-16 hours.

4. **Long-acting insulins** include glargine (Lantus) and detemir (Levemir). After subcutaneous injection, exposure of glargine's acidic solution to a neutral pH results in the formation of an insulin precipitate/depot. Detemir's longevity is due to an added fatty acid that attaches to albumin binding sites, allowing it to circulate in an inactive and reversible form until it is released at target tissues from the albumin molecule. Both glargine and detemir have a flattened peak and a dose-dependent duration of activity up to 18-24 hours. Detemir's predictable release results in a low coefficient of variation and a lower incidence of hypoglycemia. Detemir results in less weight gain than expected, perhaps because of its attachment to albumin, its ability to cross the blood-brain barrier and influence the satiety center in the hypothalamus, or due to a lower calorie intake because of less frequent and severe hypoglycemia. Although generally administered once daily, these insulins are sometimes given twice daily in type 1 diabetes, where lower doses (per kg) are utilized.

5. **Premixed insulins** are mixtures of a short-acting (regular) insulin plus NPH insulin or a fast-acting (aspart, lispro) insulin to which protamine has been added to prolong its duration of action. These insulins are typically used in a 70/30 ratio with the longer-acting

component being responsible for the majority of the effect. A ratio of 50/50 (lispro or regular plus NPH) is also available for patients whose intake of calories and carbohydrates are high.

Premixed insulins are unsuitable for use in type 1 diabetes where much greater flexibility is needed. In the type 2 insulin-requiring patient, they can be used once, twice, or three times daily. Typically a once daily evening injection is given in combination with oral agents, but the HbA$_{1c}$ target is achieved in < 50% of patients; when given as twice daily and three times daily injections, the HbA$_{1c}$ target is achieved in 60-77% of cases. Continued use of oral agents, such as metformin or TZDs, with these insulins can result in an even higher percentage of patients reaching goal. Due to lower postprandial glucose levels achieved with fast-acting insulin analogues, mixtures containing lispro or aspart are preferred over mixtures of NPH and regular insulin.

Premixed insulins also have the advantage of accuracy, as mixing of insulins by the patient results in major variations in the proportion of insulins in the syringe (Arch Int Med 1991;151:2265-9.) Therefore, mixing of insulin by the patient is potentially dangerous and should be discouraged.

Management of Glycemia in Type 2 Diabetes

A. **Initial Therapy.** Treatment algorithms for glycemic control in diabetes are difficult to create; ideally, therapy should be individualized for each patient. Nevertheless, algorithms are useful as an initial guide to therapy. Metformin should be considered as part of any regimen unless the person has a contraindication, given its low cost, its ability to help curb the weight gain that typically accompanies improved glycemic control, lack of hypoglycemia as an adverse effect, and its ability to reduce cardiovascular events and mortality. Both the ADA and the European Association for the Study of Diabetes recommend metformin as initial drug therapy for type 2 diabetes (Figure 5.2). The authors favor a more aggressive initial approach utilizing a combination of drugs to maximize

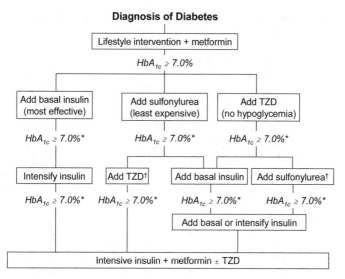

Figure 5.2. Treatment of Type 2 Diabetes: Consensus Statement from the ADA and the European Association for the Study of Diabetes

Note: This algorithm was published prior to approval of DPP-4 inhibitors. The authors favor a more aggressive approach using initial combination therapy (see Figure 5.3)

* Check HbA_{1c} every 3 months until < 7.0%, and then at least every 6 months

† Although 3 oral agents can be used, initiation/intensification of insulin is preferred based on effectiveness and expense

From: Diabetes Care 2006;29:1963-71.

glycemic control without causing severe or frequent hypoglycemia (Figure 5.3). Early upward titration (every 6 months with TZDs; every 2-4 months with other agents) and advancement to 3 or 4 drug oral therapy is recommended as needed to achieve glycemic control. In addition to pharmacologic therapy, all diabetic patients should receive medical nutritional therapy and instruction on exercise and self-monitoring of blood glucose. Aspirin, an ACE inhibitor or ARB, and a statin are also recommended in most diabetic patients to reduce overall cardiovascular risk (Chapters 6-9).

B. Insulin Therapy. When concurrent use of 3 or 4 oral agents fail to achieve adequate glycemic control, insulin therapy is required (Figure 5.4). Initially, either a once-daily basal insulin (detemir or glargine), an intermediate-acting insulin (NPH) at bedtime, or a premix at the largest meal should be added to the existing oral regimen. However, the patient should be provided with an algorithm to adjust/increase the insulin at least once a week based on the average of the blood sugars from the prior 3-5 days. The rationale for this approach is to lower fasting blood glucose to goal with insulin and maintain glycemic control throughout the day with oral agents. To optimize postprandial glycemic control, secretagogue therapy should be maintained. For once-daily insulin therapy, either premixed fixed-dose insulin containing a rapid-acting insulin (Humulog 75/25 or 50/50 or Novolog mix 70/30) can be given with the evening meal, or NPH, glargine (Lantus), or detemir (Levemir) insulin can be given at bedtime. However, with higher HbA$_{1c}$ levels (> 8.5%), it is highly unlikely that the treatment goal will be obtained with basal insulin monotherapy. Therefore, in this situation, preprandial fast-acting insulin is needed, which can be provided either with premixed insulin or with basal insulin plus fast-acting insulin. Each of the insulins used in this situation have advantages and disadvantages (Postgraduate Medicine 2006;119:8-14).

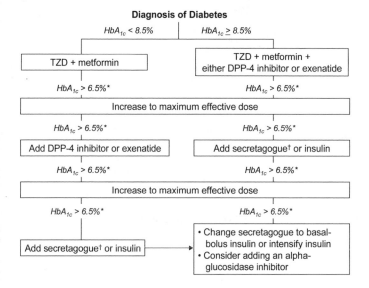

Figure 5.3. Initial Combination Therapy for Type 2 Diabetes

The authors favor a more aggressive initial approach than shown in Figure 5.2, using a combination of drugs aimed at more than one mechanism to optimize glycemic control without causing severe or frequent hypoglycemia. Lifestyle intervention should be reinforced at every visit

* Consider using a target $HbA_{1c} > 7.0\%$ (instead of 6.5%) for individuals with long-standing type 2 diabetes, significant coronary heart disease, and a predisposition to hypoglycemia (see discussion on intensive glycemic control, pp. 63-67). For initiation/titration of TZD, check HbA_{1c} at 6 months. For all other agents, check HbA_{1c} at 3 months

† Sulfonylurea or glitinide (nateglinide, repaglinide)

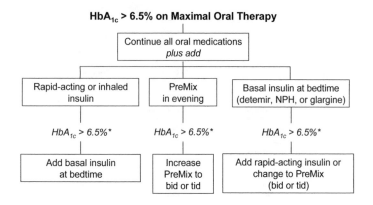

HbA₁c > 6.5% on Maximal Oral Therapy

Figure 5.4. Treatment of Type 2 Diabetes with Insulin Therapy when Oral Regimens Fail

* Check HbA₁c every 3 months.
Adapted from: Postgrad Med 2006;19:15-20.

When the HbA₁c and pre/postprandial glucose targets are not being achieved with one insulin injection per day, two or more injections are required. At this time, a fast-acting insulin should be added and secretagogues can be discontinued. If premixed insulin has been used, therapy can advance to two injections (breakfast and dinner) or three injections per day (breakfast, lunch, and dinner). If NPH, glargine, or detemir has been used, therapy can be changed to multiple injections of premixed insulin as described above; alternatively, a fast-acting insulin (lispro, aspart, or glulisine) can be added to the current bedtime regimen and administered before one or more meals to control postprandial hyperglycemia. When three or more daily insulin injections are required, then endogenous insulin production is extremely low and the patient effectively has type 1 diabetes (near complete insulin deficiency).

Special Patient Populations with Type 2 Diabetes

A. Elderly Patients. Therapeutic goals in the geriatric population should be based on the patient's functional status and underlying disease processes. A healthy geriatric patient should have the same therapeutic goals as a younger patient, including normalization of HbA_{1c}. Many elderly individuals have reduced renal function; therefore, prior to initiating or continuing metformin therapy, creatinine clearance should be ascertained. Also, many elderly patients only eat one or two meals a day, which must be taken into consideration when planning therapy, and long-acting secretagogues should not be used in this population due to erratic and/or small meals. If a secretagogue is necessary, use of a short-acting agent (repaglinide, nateglinide) should be initiated once daily, which may be sufficient, and then increased as needed to 2-3 times daily, always with meals. Because of the increased risk of hypoglycemia and the increased risk of decreased intellectual function following severe hypoglycemia in the elderly, drugs that are associated with a lower risk of hypoglycemia (metformin, TZDs, DPP-4 inhibitors, alpha-glucoside inhibitors) should be favored over secretagogues and if possible over insulin therapy.

B. Acute MI. Optimal therapy of diabetes in the setting of acute MI consists of an intravenous insulin infusion with a goal of normoglycemia followed by subcutaneous insulin therapy once the patient has stabilized and is discharged from the intensive care unit. This strategy was shown to decrease mortality at 1 year by 29% in the DIGAMI trial (J Am Coll Cardiol 1995;26:57-65). Even in patients who do not have diabetes (normal HbA_{1c} and glucose tolerance test post-discharge), elevated glucose levels are associated with a worse prognosis following MI. This is in part due to hyperglycemia-induced closure of the K^+-ATPase channels, increasing the risk of further myocardial ischemia, infarct extension, cardiac arrhythmias, congestive heart failure and death. Thus, when acute hyperglycemia occurs in the CCU, intravenous insulin is indicated to control blood sugar levels to around 100 mg/dL. Oral agents—metformin or a low-dose thiazolidinedione—may be added prior to discharge or at follow-up as appropriate, with or without stopping insulin therapy.

C. **Gestational Diabetes Mellitus (GDM).** GDM is any diabetes first recognized during pregnancy. A decrease in insulin sensitivity occurs in every pregnancy, starting in the first trimester and accelerating at the beginning of the third trimester due to increased production of human placental lactogen (HPL) by the placenta. Women with inadequate beta cell reserve manifest hyperglycemia, which is associated with adverse maternal and fetal outcomes. Thus all women at risk for diabetes should be tested for GDM in the third trimester. If diet/exercise cannot maintain preprandial and postprandial targets, then insulin therapy should be initiated. Oral hypoglycemic agents have not been approved for the treatment of GDM, though glyburide has been shown to be effective without having adverse fetal effects in a clinical trial (N Eng J Med 2000;343:1134-8). Although several oral agents have been labeled as Category B in pregnancy, metformin is the standard of care, and the use of other oral agents is not recommended. Women taking metformin at the time they become pregnant can continue the drug at least through the first trimester, and perhaps throughout pregnancy. However, initiation of metformin during pregnancy is not currently recommended. Of the sulfonylureas, only glyburide has been used before and during pregnancy; controlled trials are needed to determine whether glyburide is safe in early pregnancy or effective later in gestation, and other sulfonylureas should be withdrawn and replaced with insulin. There are no data using thiazolidinediones in pregnancy so they should be discontinued prior to conception and stopped if a woman discovers she is pregnant. A consensus statement for the medical care of pregnant women with preexisting diabetes has been published (Diabetes Care 2008;31:1060-79).

D. **Severe/Frequent Hypoglycemia.** These patients require evaluation by a diabetes specialist to determine if the problem is related to insulin dosing errors or hypoglycemia unawareness. Hypoglycemia unawareness occurs as a result of recurrent hypoglycemic episodes, as hypoglycemic events that occur within 3 days of a prior episode are associated with less catecholamine production, leaving only symptoms of neuroglycopenia to warn the patient to correct the hypoglycemia. One strategy to attempt to resume the ability to sense hypoglycemia is to allow the sugars to run in the range of 200-300 mg/dL for a few weeks followed by cautious and gradual resumption of intensive glucose control. In this way, hypothalamic sensitization to hypoglycemia may be restored. Conversion to a continuous subcutaneous insulin infusion using a pump may resolve this problem. Islet cell/whole pancreas transplantation is also a consideration.

Chapter 6

Prevention and Treatment of Complications of Type 2 Diabetes

The underlying pathophysiology of both microvascular and macrovascular complications of diabetes is chronic exposure of non-insulin sensitive tissues to hyperglycemia. The presence of a large glucose flux stimulates rarely used metabolic pathways, and enzymes such as aldose reductase, hexokinase, and protein kinase C-β (PKC$_\beta$) are activated. As a result, substances such as sorbitol and glucosamine accumulate in the cytoplasm, which may cause osmotic swelling of cells. Furthermore, the functioning of key proteins is disrupted by irreversible glycosylation. These perturbations increase oxidative stress, which in turn leads to decreased nitric oxide levels, endothelial dysfunction, and further tissue damage. This endothelial damage to major arteries and capillaries leads to an increased frequency of macrovascular complications (coronary artery disease, cerebrovascular disease, peripheral vascular disease) and microvascular complications (retinopathy, neuropathy, nephropathy). In addition, tissues with potentially high levels of aldose reductase activity, such as the nerve and lens of the eye, can accumulate excess sorbitol, resulting in neuropathy and cataracts, respectively.

The prevention of chronic hyperglycemia in type 2 diabetes will prevent, ameliorate, or delay the complications of diabetes (Table 6.1). This chapter reviews strategies to both treat and prevent the macrovascular and microvascular complications of diabetes.

Macrovascular Disease and Diabetes

A. Overview. Diabetes predisposes to a variety of circulatory disturbances—diffuse accelerated atherosclerosis, a prothrombotic state, endothelial dysfunction, autonomic neuropathy—that increase the risk of coronary artery disease (angina, acute MI, sudden death), heart failure, cerebrovascular disease (TIA, cerebral infarction), and peripheral arterial disease (claudication, gangrene, foot ulcers, leg amputation). All of these are dramatically increased in active smokers. Cardiomyopathy and orthostatic hypotension can also cause significant disability.

1. **Cardiovascular disease.** Cardiovascular disease is responsible for 75% of all deaths in diabetes, and diabetic subjects without coronary disease have as high a risk of MI as nondiabetic subjects who have already had an MI (Table 6.2). Diabetic subjects are at increased risk of silent myocardial ischemia and infarction, and up to one-third of diabetic patients with acute MI do not manifest chest pain. One-month mortality rates following acute MI are increased by 50% in diabetic patients, and by 5 years, cumulative mortality is 50%, twice the rate found in nondiabetic patients. Diabetes is also the most important risk factor for the development of congestive heart failure following acute MI. Diabetic patients also have a higher incidence of atrial and ventricular fibrillation. Following balloon angioplasty, diabetic patients have more restenosis, more repeat revascularization procedures, and reduced long-term survival. Following CABG, diabetic patients have more in-hospital deaths and strokes, more late MI and revascularization procedures, and reduced long-term survival (approximately 25% of diabetic patients die within 5 years of CABG). The risk of heart failure in persons with diabetes is increased 2-fold in men and 5-fold in women.

2. **Cerebrovascular disease.** The risk of cerebral infarction is increased 3- to 10-fold in diabetic patients, and individuals with diabetes have increased morbidity and mortality following a stroke, which is proportional to the serum glucose level at the time of the event. Diabetic patients are also less likely to be discharged to home than to a chronic care facility and less likely to return to work.

3. **Peripheral arterial disease.** Compared to nondiabetic subjects, the risk of peripheral arterial disease is increased 4-fold in diabetic men and 30-fold in diabetic women, and risk is further increased in active smokers. Peripheral arterial disease also manifests at an earlier age in persons with diabetes. In the U.S., 17% of individuals with diabetes have peripheral arterial disease, and diabetes is responsible for more than 50,000 lower extremity amputations each year, making

Table 6.1. Prevention/Treatment of Diabetes-Related Complications

Complication	Screening	Prevention/Treatment
Cardiovascular disease	• Screen annually for cardiac risk factors* • Exercise stress test for high-risk individuals† • Ankle/brachial index	• Antiplatelet, ACEI or ARB, statin • Control cardiac risk factors* • Revascularization of high-grade arterial stenoses
Retinopathy	• Annual ophthalmoscopy exam through dilated pupil	• Tight control of glycemia/BP • Laser photocoagulation for nonproliferative retinopathy (severe), proliferative retinopathy, macular edema
Nephropathy	• Screen for microalbuminuria and renal function	• Tight control of glycemia/BP • ACEI and/or ARB • Possible protein restriction • Referral to nephrologist for GFR < 60 cc/min/1.73m²
Neuropathy	• Annual foot examination	• Tight control of glycemia • Foot care instruction • Specific measures based on peripheral/autonomic neuropathy
Foot ulcers	• Self-examination for foot trauma • Annual foot examination	• Well-fitted shoes, callus debridement, proper foot/nail care • Antibiotics ± debridement for infected ulcers • Revascularization of high-grade arterial stenoses
Infections	–	• Influenza/pneumococcal vaccines • Consider hepatitis vaccinations

DKA, hyperosmolar coma, hypoglycemia (see text), screen for hepatitis

ACEI = ACE inhibitor, ARB = angiotensin receptor blocker, BP = blood pressure, GFR = glomerular filtration rate

* Hypertension, dyslipidemia, physical inactivity, overweight/obesity, tobacco use, micro/macroalbuminuria; review family history

† Cardiac symptoms, abnormal ECG, peripheral arterial or cerebrovascular disease, sedentary lifestyle plus age > 35 prior to starting a vigorous exercise program, or 2 or more cardiac risk factors

Table 6.2. Incidence of Myocardial Infarction at 7 Years

	No Prior MI	Prior MI
Diabetes	20%	45%
No diabetes	3%	19%

it the leading cause of non-traumatic amputation. Amputation is usually caused by a foot ulcer that fails to heal and then becomes infected, ischemic, and often gangrenous. Since diabetic subjects often have reduced sensation in their feet (loss of protective sensation) and impaired wound healing (Lancet 2005;366:1736-43), even a simple cut or callus may go undetected until the late stages of infection when amputation is required. Arterial stenoses in diabetic patients are more likely to be distal in location (tibial, peroneal arteries), making it difficult for collaterals to form and making the lesions less amenable to revascularization. (The distal location results in a lower prevalence of claudication in diabetic compared to nondiabetic patients with peripheral arterial disease.) Active use of tobacco limits patency following revascularization.

B. **Treatment of Macrovascular Disease.** Chapters 4-9 detail measures to reduce cardiovascular risk in type 2 diabetes, including therapeutic lifestyle changes (diet, physical activity, weight control, smoking cessation), control of hypertension and dyslipidemia, and use of aspirin, ARBs/ACE inhibitors, and statins. When percutaneous revascularization is required, intensive antiplatelet therapy including a glycoprotein IIb/IIIa inhibitor is associated with improved outcomes. The role of intensive glycemic therapy on macrovascular complications is described in Chapter 5. Combination therapy using aspirin, a statin, an ACE inhibitor or ARB, and a beta-blocker could reduce the risk of death, MI, and stroke by 75% (Table 6.3). For patients with symptomatic claudication, cilostazol (preferred) or pentoxifylline may improve symptoms and functional capacity. For critical limb ischemia, revascularization and sometimes amputation is required.

Table 6.3. ASAB-*ASAP!* Reducing Cardiovascular Events in Type 2 Diabetes

Measure	Relative Risk Reduction
Aspirin*	~ 25%
Statin†	~ 25%
ACE inhibitor or ARB‡	~ 25%
Beta or calcium **B**locker¶	~ 25%
Cumulative relative risk reduction	~ 75%
Number of events (death, MI, stroke) prevented in 1000 diabetic patients¥	1 event prevented every 12 days

ARB = angiotensin receptor blocker, ASAP = as soon as possible. Type 2 diabetes is associated with a cluster of cardiovascular risk factors (hypertension, dyslipidemia, insulin resistance, prothrombotic state, endothelial dysfunction) that require treatment to optimize cardiovascular prognosis. Only 20% of diabetic patients meet any of the major national guidelines for control of glucose, hemoglobin A_{1c}, cholesterol, or blood pressure. Appropriate drug therapy could reduce the risk of death, MI, and stroke by 75%.

* Aspirin 81-325 mg/d. Consider adding clopidogrel (75 mg/d) to aspirin in high risk individuals or substituting it for aspirin in aspirin-intolerant patients.

† Statin (e.g., atorvastatin 10 mg/d, simvastatin 40 mg/d) to reduce LDL-C by *at least 30-40%*, regardless of baseline LDL-C. A minimum LDL-C target < 100 mg/dL is recommended. For patients with CHD or other clinical forms of atherosclerosis, it is reasonable to treat to an LDL-C , 70 mg/dL. High-dose statin ± adjunctive drug therapy may be required to reach LDL-C target.

‡ Consider ACE inhibitor in patients with hypertension, atherosclerotic vascular disease, or age ≥ 55 years with ≥ 1 other risk factor (hypertension, elevated total cholesterol, low HDL cholesterol, cigarette smoking, microalbuminuria). For patients with hypertension or proteinuria or intolerance to ACE inhibitors, an ARB can be used as an alternative.

¶ Consider beta blocker in diabetic patients with hypertension, LV dysfunction, prior MI, or high sympathetic tone (resting heart rate > 90 bpm). Carvedilol is a beta blocker with alpha-1 blockade that improves insulin resistance; beta blockers without alpha blockade may worsen insulin resistance. The addition of a low-dose thiazide diuretic (to an ARB or ACE inhibitor) followed by a beta blocker or calcium blocker may be required to achieve/maintain BP < 130/80 mmHg.

¥ Assumes annual event rate of 4%. Use of all 4 therapies in high-risk individuals would reduce annual risk to about 1%. This translates into 570,000 deaths, MIs, or strokes prevented each year among 19 million diabetic patients in the U.S. Smoking cessation, diet modification, weight control, and increased physical activity further reduce risk.

From: Freed, MS, and O'Keefe, Jr, JH. Additional references: Lancet 2002;360:2-3, BMJ 2003;326:1419-24.

Diabetic Retinopathy

A. **Overview.** Diabetes is the leading cause of blindness in adults aged 20-74 years, causing more than 15,000 new cases each year in the U.S. alone. Visual loss can occur in several ways: (1) increased capillary permeability can lead to macular edema; (2) new blood vessels that grow on the posterior surface of the vitreous in response to retinal ischemia can rupture and cause vitreous hemorrhage; (3) new blood vessels can pull on sections of the retina and cause retinal detachment; and (4) neovascularization on the iris associated with proliferative retinopathy can cause vision-threatening glaucoma. It has recently been hypothesized that degeneration of neural tissue in the retina precedes and results in the development of microvascular changes. Diabetic retinopathy progresses in stages from nonproliferative (background) retinopathy to proliferative retinopathy, and both eyes are usually affected at the same time. *Nonproliferative retinopathy* is characterized by increased capillary permeability, capillary closure and dilatation, microaneurysms, scar (retinitis proliferans), arteriovenous shunts, dilated veins, hemorrhages (dot and blot), cotton-wool spots (retinal infarcts), and hard exudates due to leakage of fat and protein from permeable capillaries. Nonproliferative retinopathy does not result in loss of vision unless leakage from permeable capillaries occurs in the macular area. *Proliferative retinopathy* is characterized by new blood vessel formation, vitreous hemorrhage and retinal detachment, and is more common in patients receiving insulin. A sudden increase in the number of cotton-wool spots (microinfarcts) may signal the onset of progressive retinopathy; this complication should be suspected when impaired vision is not corrected by glasses. Retinopathy eventually affects about 85% of individuals with diabetes and is present in up to 20% of patients at the time of diagnosis. Among diabetic patients with nonproliferative retinopathy, 10%-15% will progress to proliferative retinopathy within 10 years, and half of these individuals will develop blindness within 5 years. Other eye problems associated with diabetes include cataracts and glaucoma. Blurred vision due to increased sorbitol content of the lens secondary to prolonged hyperglycemia can develop during rapid changes in blood glucose levels in the absence of retinopathy and may take several weeks to resolve after the hyperglycemia is corrected. Vision changes can also lead to insulin errors so it is important to ask patients about their vision.

B. Treatment. Diabetic retinopathy is often asymptomatic until visual loss develops, and laser photocoagulation can slow or prevent vision loss. Therefore, retinal evaluation through a dilated pupil by an ophthalmologist is recommended for all diabetic patients at the time of diagnosis and on an annual basis; referral to a retinal specialist is required when retinopathy develops.

1. **Control of glycemia and blood pressure.** Compared to conventional therapy, better glycemic control reduced the risk of microvascular complications, including retinopathy, by 25% in UKPDS. In the same study, tight blood pressure control reduced the progression of retinopathy by 34%. In the Diabetes Control and Complications Trial (DCCT) of type 1 diabetes, a significant difference in HbA$_{1c}$ of 2.1% resulted in a 76% decrease in the onset of retinopathy and a 54% reduction in progression in those with retinopathy at initiation of therapy (N Engl J Med 1993;329:977-86).

2. **Laser therapy.** Laser photocoagulation significantly reduced severe vision loss in the Early Treatment Diabetic Retinopathy Study (ETDRS) and is recommend for diabetic subjects with severe nonproliferative retinopathy, proliferative retinopathy, or macular edema. Photocoagulation destroys peripheral retinal tissue to prevent ischemia in vital retinal areas such as the macula. While visual acuity is preserved, peripheral vision, night vision and color discrimination (the functions of the peripheral retina) are compromised. Vitrectomy is indicated for vitreous hemorrhage or retinal detachment.

Diabetic Nephropathy

A. Overview. Diabetic nephropathy develops in 25% of patients with type 2 diabetes and is responsible for 50% of end-stage renal disease (ESRD) in the U.S. The risk of progression to ESRD is highest in Native Americans, Mexican Americans, and African Americans.

1. **Types of diabetic nephropathy.** Two distinct forms of diabetic

nephropathy exist, which may or may not be present at the same time. *Diffuse disease* is the most common form and consists of generalized mesangial thickening and widening of the glomerular basement membrane. *Nodular disease* is characterized by large accumulations of periodic acid-Schiff-positive material at the periphery of the glomerular tufts, with or without hyalinization of arterioles, fibrin caps, and glomerular occlusion.

2. **Progression of Diabetic Nephropathy.** Regardless of form, diabetic nephropathy may be "silent" for 10-15 years and commonly progresses in stages:

   a. **Hyperfiltration of kidneys.** Hyperglycemia leads to an increase in renal blood flow, hyperfiltration, and increased glomerular pressure. Because of this, the glomerular filtration rate (GFR) may be 40% or more above normal in the early stages of the disease.

   b. **Appearance of microalbuminuria.** Microalbuminuria is defined as urinary albumin excretion 30-299 mg/24 h (or 30-299 mcg/mg creatinine on a spot collection). Microalbuminuria, as well as being the earliest warning sign for diabetic nephropathy, is also associated with increased cardiovascular mortality and is an indication for screening for atherosclerotic vascular disease and aggressive risk factor modification. Microalbuminuria can be a marker of generalized endothelial dysfunction since the glomerulus is an arteriole and therefore can act as a "window" to the vasculature. All persons with type 2 diabetes should be tested for microalbuminuria at the time of diagnosis and annually thereafter by an albumin-to-creatinine ratio in a spot urine. Positive tests with reagent-tablets or dipstick should be confirmed using another test. While 80% of type 1 diabetic subjects with microalbuminuria will progress to macroalbuminuria within 10 years if untreated, this only occurs in 25% of type 2 microalbuminuric subjects. Kidney biopsy in type 2 diabetes shows classic changes of diabetic nephropathy in one-third, vascular changes in one-third, and a normal biopsy in the remaining one-third of subjects.

c. **Onset of macroalbuminuria** (urinary albumin excretion ≥ 300 mg/24 h or ≥ 300 mcg/mg creatinine on a spot collection).

d. **Decline in GFR.** Once macroalbuminuria begins, renal function if left untreated typically declines at a rate of approximately 1 cc/min/month. Azotemia usually begins 2-3 years after macroalbuminuria is detected. Deterioration in renal function is accelerated by concomitant hypertension.

e. **Progression to end-stage renal disease.** Only 20% of diabetic subjects with nephropathy progress to dialysis or transplant since the majority succumb to cardiovascular disease before end-stage renal disease develops. Progression to end-stage renal disease is more common in type 1 diabetes than in type 2 diabetes.

B. **Treatment.** Interventions aimed at slowing the progression of diabetic nephropathy include: tight glycemic control (nephropathy reduced by 21% in ADVANCE, p. 65); aggressive blood pressure control, including use of a renin-angiotensin system (RAS) inhibitor (ACE inhibitor, ARB, direct renin inhibitor); and possibly protein restriction (≤ 0.8 gm/kg body weight/day) at the onset of overt nephropathy. Patients receiving ACE inhibitors or ARBs should be monitored for hyperkalemia and azotemia, and these agents are contraindicated during the prepregnancy period and during pregnancy (Chapter 7). The goal of therapy, particularly in the setting of microalbuminuria, is to reduce urine albumin levels to the normal range. Nondihydropyridine calcium antagonists and/or beta-blockers can be used for patients intolerant to ACE inhibitors/ARBs. The blood pressure goal in patients with diabetic nephropathy is ≤ 120/75 mmHg. Referral to a nephrologist is recommended for patients with GFR < 60 cc/min/1.73m^2. Patients should be instructed to promptly report symptoms of urinary tract infection (dysuria, frequency, hematuria, fever, chills, flank or lower abdominal pain/pressure).

Diabetic Neuropathy

Persons with type 2 diabetes are at increased risk of developing peripheral and autonomic neuropathies. *Peripheral polyneuropathy* is associated with sensory symptoms such as numbness, pain, and hyperesthesias. Most patients with diabetic neuropathic pain will require drug therapy (e.g., clonazepam, nortriptyline, tramadol, pregabalin [Lyrica], duloxetine [Cymbalta], amitriptyline, capsaicin cream). *Mononeuropathy* can also occur and manifests as sudden onset of wrist drop, foot drop, or cranial nerve paralysis (III, IV, VI, VII). Spontaneous remission almost always occurs over a 6-12 week period due to revascularization of the nerve. Infrequently, *radiculopathy* can develop, and when it involves one or more dermatomes in the chest wall or abdomen, it can mimic acute myocardial infarction, herpes zoster, or an acute abdomen. Radiculopathy almost invariably resolves. *Autonomic neuropathy* can affect many organs and result in a variety of abnormalities, including esophageal dysmotility, bladder dysfunction/paralysis, erectile dysfunction, gastroparesis with delayed gastric emptying and early satiety, small bowel dysfunction (diabetic diarrhea), Charcot's joint (dislocation/collapse of one or more joints or bones in foot), abnormal sweat production (anhidrosis or hyperhidrosis), and cardiac dysfunction (orthostatic hypotension, tachycardia). Tight glucose control can slow/prevent the development of diabetic neuropathy. Patients with peripheral neuropathy should take special precautions during exercise (Chapter 4) and require special attention to foot care. *Entrapment neuropathies* such as carpal tunnel syndrome, ulnar entrapment at the elbow, meralgia paresthetica, and foot drop due to common peroneal palsy are more common with diabetes. Reasons for this include excess collagen production (from protein glycosylation) and increased vulnerability of the diabetic nerve to external pressure. A rare neuropathy is *diabetic amyotrophy*, which presents with severe pain and weakness of the quadriceps muscles. Most often this syndrome occurs in men with recent onset of mild diabetes and a history of excessive alcohol intake. Electrophysiological studies demonstrate some features of an alcoholic myopathy. Pain management for up to one year and physical therapy to improve muscle strength are the cornerstones of therapy.

Diabetic Foot Ulcers

Due to "clawing" of the neuropathic foot, which is caused by weakness of the interossei and excess pressure on the metatarsal heads accompanying a loss of protective sensation, ulceration of the plantar surface of the foot may occur (Lancet 2005;366:1736-43). The frequent coexistence of peripheral arterial disease and impaired wound healing contribute to the development and progression of ulcers, which are frequently complicated by polymicrobial infection. Measures to reduce the development and progression of foot ulcers include the use of well-fitting walking shoes with extra depth, molded insoles, and a "rocker bottom" sole; callus debridement; revascularization for significant peripheral arterial disease (J Am Coll Cardiol 2006;47:921-9); and patient education about the need for daily foot monitoring, proper foot and nail care, and selection of appropriate footwear. Treatment of foot ulcers requires adequate antimicrobial therapy, debridement, and complete absence of weight bearing so that the ulcer can heal from the base. To achieve healing and avoid weight bearing, contact casting or a protective boot may be needed since most patients are not compliant with complete bed rest. When an ulcer is failing to heal, vascular insufficiency or underlying osteomyelitis should be considered and treated appropriately. Unfortunately, the diagnosis of osteomyelitis may require a bone biopsy because changes in x-rays/bone scan caused by increased blood flow secondary to arteriovenous shunting from autonomic neuropathy can mimic osteomyelitis.

Infection

Urinary tract and skin infections are especially common and more severe in diabetic patients, possibly due to impaired leukocyte function. Patients with diabetes are also predisposed to several types of unusual infections. *Rhinocerebral mucormycosis* is a fungal infection that usually develops during or after an episode of diabetic ketoacidosis. Manifestations include sudden periorbital swelling with bloody nasal discharge and black, necrotic nasal mucosa. Cranial nerve palsies and cavernous sinus thrombosis can occur and signify a poor prognosis. This condition may present as failure to wake from coma upon treatment of diabetic ketoacidosis. Treatment consists of antifungal therapy and emergency surgical debridement. Without prompt intervention, death usually occurs within 2 weeks. *Malignant external otitis* presents with severe ear pain, fever, leukocytosis, and ear drainage and is often caused by Pseudomonas aeruginosa infecting a relatively ischemic "watershed" area of the external auditory canal. Cranial nerve palsies can occur, and facial nerve involvement is associated with a 50% mortality rate. Treatment consists of urgent debridement plus broad-spectrum antibiotics. *Emphysematous cholecystitis* presents with right upper quadrant pain, fever, and gas in the gallbladder wall on flat plate of the abdomen. Gas-producing organisms other than clostridia are frequently present, and this condition is associated with a higher incidence of gallbladder gangrene and perforation than typical cholecystitis. *Emphysematous pyelonephritis* is diagnosed by gas in the kidney or perirenal space in a patient with pyelonephritis. *Perinephric abscess* is also more common in the diabetic patient. Antibiotics are often ineffective, and surgical drainage or nephrectomy may be required. Mortality rates may be as high as 80%. *Necrotizing fasciitis* is an infection that rapidly spreads through the tissue planes of the abdominal wall and is usually secondary to a trivial infection. Treatment consists of urgent antimicrobial therapy and surgical debridement of necrotic tissue. Mortality rates are extremely high.

Diabetic Ketoacidosis

Diabetic ketoacidosis (DKA) is a medical emergency that can progress rapidly to coma and death without prompt treatment. DKA develops when, with very low insulin levels, the body is unable to metabolize glucose and instead breaks down fat for energy, resulting in the accumulation of ketones (acetoacetate, beta-hydroxybutyrate, acetone) in the blood. DKA is much more common in type 1 diabetes, where it can occur spontaneously and may be the initial manifestation of diabetes, but it can also develop in people with type 2 diabetes following acute physical stress (infection, surgery, myocardial infarction), emotional stress, prolonged hyperglycemia, or after discontinuation of insulin therapy. Symptoms usually consist of excessive urination and thirst, nausea, vomiting, and abdominal pain due to ketosis.

Affected individuals often present with very rapid and shallow breathing due to acidosis and have a fruity smell to their breath (like nail polish remover). An anion gap metabolic acidosis is present and often severe. DKA is treated with intravenous insulin, fluids and electrolytes, gradual reduction of blood sugar, occasional small doses of bicarbonate for severe acidosis, and treatment of intercurrent illness (e.g., infection, MI). There are many possible protocols; one is shown in Table 6.4. All patients with unexplained DKA and type 2 diabetes should have an ECG and troponin levels checked to exclude an MI.

Hyperosmolar Coma

This serious complication usually develops in elderly type 2 diabetic patients following an acute illness (e.g., infection, stroke) or following institution of peritoneal dialysis or diuretic therapy. Hyperosmolar coma may be the initial presentation of type 2 diabetes. The predominant pathophysiology is severe dehydration so that the kidney cannot excrete glucose, resulting in serum glucose levels that often reach extreme levels (> 1000 mg/dL). The most common symptom is increasing lethargy, which can progress to loss of consciousness over a period of days. Treatment consists of intravenous fluids and electrolytes, gradual reduction of blood glucose levels, and treatment of intercurrent illness. The prognosis is far worse than that of DKA, and the vast majority of patients who recover do not need insulin to control their diabetes.

Hypoglycemia

Hypoglycemia usually occur in diabetic subjects who have taken excessive insulin or insulin secretagogues. Severe hypoglycemia is extremely rare with metformin, thiazolidinediones, DPP-4 inhibitors, incretin mimetics, amylin analogs, or alpha-glucosidase inhibitors when not used in combination with insulin or sulfonylureas. Adrenergic symptoms include sweating, tremor, palpitations, and weakness. If adrenergic symptoms are missed or ignored, neuroglycopenia can occur and present as irritability, confusion, double vision, slurred speech, or coma. If hypoglycemia is prolonged/severe, seizures, accidental injury, and irreversible brain damage can occur. Importantly, severe hypoglycemia induces a marked increase in sympathetic tone, which can trigger acute MI or sudden cardiac arrest, particularly in patients with long-standing diabetes and advanced atherosclerosis. When hypoglycemia occurs frequently (less than 3 days between episodes), "hypoglycemic unawareness" may develop, as hypothalamic neurons, which are dependent on glucose crossing the blood-brain barrier, adapt to hypoglycemia by increasing the activity of the K^+-ATPase channels to preserve intraneuronal energy. As a result, hypoglycemia fails to initiate through-signals from these cells and catecholamine production, leading to lack of awareness and failure to correct the hypoglycemia. The hypothalamic neurons can be resensitized to hypoglycemia by allowing hyperglycemia to persist for several days at a level that avoids hypoglycemic episodes from occurring. In this way, hypoglycemic unawareness can often be corrected. Hypoglycemic episodes are treated by sugar-containing foods, intravenous glucose, or glucagon to raise blood sugar levels. Special therapeutic considerations for patients with frequent/severe hypoglycemia are described in Chapter 5.

Other Complications of Diabetes

Persons with diabetes are predisposed to *fatty infiltration of the liver* and to a variety of *skin disorders*, including necrobiosis lipoidica diabeticorum (plaque with central yellowish area and brownish border over the anterior legs with or without ulceration); diabetic dermopathy (small rounded raised plaques over the anterior tibial surface); bullous diabeticorum (uncommon; bullae may be hemorrhagic or clear); skin infections with Candida and dermatophytes; bacterial infections; vaginal moniliasis; atrophy of adipose tissue (at site of insulin injections), which is rare with human insulin; hypertrophy of fat; scleredema (common benign thickening of skin over shoulders and upper back); Dupuytren's contractions of joints; and frozen shoulder.

Table 6.4. Guidelines for Management of Diabetic Ketoacidosis

Establish diagnosis
- Measure serum glucose and ketones and arterial blood gas
- Obtain complete blood cell count, serum electrolytes, renal profile (BUN, creatinine)
- Obtain fresh-voided urine sample for urinalysis
- Record pulse, blood pressure (lying/sitting, if possible), respiratory rate, temperature
- Eliminate other causes of acidosis (uremia, alcoholism, salicylate overdose)

If ketoacidosis is confirmed¶
- Admit to diabetes unit
- Give 10 U regular insulin intravenously immediately
- Start normal saline infusion at 500 mL/hr IV for first 2 hours then 200 mL/hr*
- Add 100 U regular insulin to 500 mL saline solution. Dispose of first 50 mL through tubing. Piggyback to IV line and infuse at 0.5 mL/kg/hr
- Obtain electrocardiogram and institute cardiac monitoring when appropriate
- Measure serum potassium level; if < 5.5 mEq/L and there is reasonable urine output, add potassium chloride 20 mEq/L

Monitor hourly to:
- Adjust insulin. Infuse 5 mL/hr to maintain decrease in serum glucose at 50-150 mg/dL per hour and to keep serum glucose > 250 mg/dL until hydration improves
- Record vital signs and determine fluid input/output†
- Measure glucose level
- Test all urine for ketones (hourly if catheter is in situ)‡

Monitor every 2 hours for serum glucose, electrolytes, renal profile
Monitor every 6 hours for serum magnesium and serum phosphate

When serum glucose falls below 250 mg/dL
- Change IV to 5% dextrose in normal saline solution and run at 150 mL/hr. Reduce insulin infusion by 50%

When serum glucose is below 250 mg/dL, serum and urine are free of ketones, and electrolytes are normal
- Start an ADA diet and administer short-or fast-acting insulin subcutaneously before meals and NPH or glargine insulin at bedtime. Discontinue IV fluids and IV insulin 1-2 hours after first insulin injection. Continue to monitor glucose every 2 hours

---

¶ Correct precipitating event, if present (e.g., infection, GI bleed, PE, MI). Be aware of severe/uncommon complications (DVT, PE, MI, ARDS, cerebral edema, infection, etc.)

* Patients with severe hypotension/hypovolemia may require higher infusion rates. Monitor for signs of heart failure in patients with LV dysfunction.

† An indwelling urinary catheter is seldom needed and increases the risk of infection.

‡ The level of measured ketones may increase during clinical improvement. This is due to a shift from beta-hydroxybutyrate production to the less acidic acetoacetate or acetone bodies, giving the false impression that the ketotic state is getting worse.

Chapter 7

Control of Dyslipidemia in Type 2 Diabetes

Overview of Diabetic Dyslipidemia

A. **Introduction.** Elevated plasma levels of total cholesterol and LDL cholesterol (LDL-C) and low plasma levels of HDL cholesterol (HDL-C) are major modifiable lipid risk factors for atherothrombotic vascular disease. It has been estimated that for each 1% decrease in LDL-C and each 1% increase in HDL-C, the risk for cardiovascular events falls by 2% and 3%, respectively. Dramatic results from the Collaborative Atorvastatin Diabetes Study (CARDS) and the Heart Protection Study (HPS) have shown that statins reduce major cardiovascular events by 25-37% and stroke by 13-48% in patients with type 2 diabetes, including subjects with "normal" LDL-C levels (Tables 7.1, 7.2). Optimization of the lipid profile is the *single most important intervention* for improving cardiovascular prognosis in type 2 diabetes, reducing the risk of coronary death, MI, stroke, and revascularization procedures. In Steno-2, 70% of the 47% reduction in cardiovascular risk attributable to intensive multifactorial intervention was due to improvements in lipid profile (N Engl J Med 2003;348:383-93).

B. **Lipid Profile.** Diabetic dyslipidemia is characterized by elevated triglycerides (≥ 150 mg/dL), depressed HDL-C (< 40 mg/dL), and elevated small dense LDL-C particles, which are easily oxidized and highly atherogenic since they more readily attach to the scavenger receptor on the macrophage and more easily enter the subintimal space. This atherogenicity is amplified if the LDL-C particles are also glycosylated due to chronic hyperglycemia. LDL-C levels are generally normal to moderately elevated and no different than levels in nondiabetic patients. Patients with diabetic dyslipidemia often have rapid progression of CHD due to highly atherogenic LDL-C particles, prothrombogenic hemostatic function (impaired fibrinolysis, activated platelets and Factor

VIII), and endothelial dysfunction. It has been estimated that diabetic dyslipidemia confers a cardiovascular risk similar to an LDL-C level of 150-220 mg/dL (Circulation 1997;95:1-4).

C. **Lipid Therapy and the New CHD Paradigm.** It has now been established that the most dangerous (i.e., rupture-prone) atherosclerotic plaques are not necessarily those causing the most severe narrowing, and that most acute coronary syndromes are caused by lesions that were less than 70% stenotic (nonobstructive) prior to ulceration, rupture, and thrombosis. Nonobstructive plaques with extensive inflammation (stimulated by oxidized lipoproteins in the vessel wall), lipid-rich cores, and thin fibrous caps are more prone to ulceration and rupture than long-standing obstructive lesions with extensive calcification and thick fibrous caps comprised of dense collagenous tissue.

Moderate reductions in LDL-C slow the progression of coronary artery disease in most patients, and lesion regression is more frequent with LDL-C reduction. Nevertheless, the beneficial effects of lipid therapy are due more to plaque stabilization than to changes in stenosis severity, which are generally modest and disproportionate to the 25-50% reduction in major cardiovascular events. Plaque stabilization, which can be accomplished in weeks to months with aggressive treatment of dyslipidemia, may be related to resorption of macrophage and extracellular lipid deposits, a decrease in neointimal inflammation, and maintenance of fibrous cap integrity. Effective treatment transforms the inflamed, friable plaque into a stable, fibrotic plaque that is less prone to ulceration, rupture, and thrombosis. In addition, lipid-modifying drug therapy improves endothelial dysfunction caused by dyslipidemia, resulting in additional vasodilatory, antithrombotic, and anti-inflammatory effects. Treatment of dyslipidemia and other concomitant risk factors is essential to improving long-term cardiovascular prognosis in type 2 diabetes.

Intensive LDL Lowering and
Cardiovascular Prognosis: Lower is Better

A. **Overview.** Recent, large-scale, randomized trials have demonstrated improved cardiovascular prognosis through intensive LDL-C lowering, prompting the National Cholesterol Education Program (NCEP) Adult Treatment Panel (ATP) III and the American Heart Association (AHA)/American College of Cardiology (ACC) to issue guideline updates recommending expanded and more intensive use of lipid-modifying drug therapy, particularly statins (Circulation 2004;110:227-239, Circulation 2006;113:2363-2372). Data from epidemiological studies and clinical trials have shown that for every 1 mg/dL reduction in LDL, the relative risk for CHD is reduced by 1% (Figure 7.1). Benefits extend to LDL-C levels of 50-70 mg/dL, well below the previously recommended LDL-C target of < 100 mg/dL for high-risk patients. Average cholesterol levels in the U.S. are nearly twice the normal physiological level (Figure 7.2).

B. **Dyslipidemia Trials in the General Population** (see pp. 115-116 for dyslipidemia trials in type 2 diabetic subjects)

1. **Placebo-Controlled Trials.** A meta-analysis of more than 30 trials using diet, drugs, or surgery to lower cholesterol has shown that for every 1% total cholesterol is lowered, total mortality is reduced by 1.1% (Circulation 1995;91:2274-82; Circulation 1998;97:946-52). Statins are overwhelmingly the drug class of choice for improving dyslipidemia and cardiovascular prognosis. In addition to lowering LDL-C levels by 18-55%, they also reduce the number of small, dense (atherogenic) LDL-C particles, raise HDL-C levels by 5-10%, and lower triglycerides by 7-30%. When CHD event rates are plotted against LDL-C levels, a direct relationship is apparent, without a lower threshold, in both primary and secondary prevention trials (Figures 7.3, 7.4). In the Heart Protection Study (HPS), the largest statin study to date, 20,536 patients with arterial occlusive disease or diabetes were

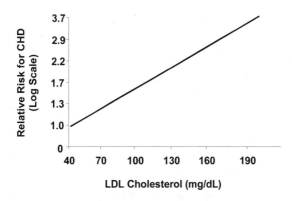

Figure 7.1. Relationship Between LDL Cholesterol Levels and Relative Risk for CHD

The log-linear relationship between LDL-C and CHD risk is consistent with a large body of data from epidemiological studies and clinical trials. For every 30 mg/dL change in LDL-C, the relative risk for CHD is changed in proportion by about 30%. The relative risk is set at 1.0 for LDL-C = 40 mg/dL. From: NCEP ATP III guideline update (Circulation 2004;110:227-239).

randomized to simvastatin 40 mg/d or placebo. At 5 years, simvastatin reduced the risk of coronary death by 18% (5.7% vs. 6.9%, p = 0.0005) (Lancet 2002;360:7-22). Patients with baseline LDL-C < 100 mg/dL (~ 70 mg/dL or less on treatment) had the same relative risk reduction as patients with baseline LDL-C > 100 mg/dL. In the Anglo-Scandinavian Cardiac Outcomes Trial (ASCOT) (Lancet 2003;361:1149) and the Collaborative Atorvastatin Diabetes Study (CARDS) (Lancet 2004;364:685-96), statins reduced the risk of CHD by 25-37% compared to placebo. In these studies, statin therapy was well tolerated and extremely safe: muscle and liver side effects were similar to placebo and rhabdomyolysis was very rare.

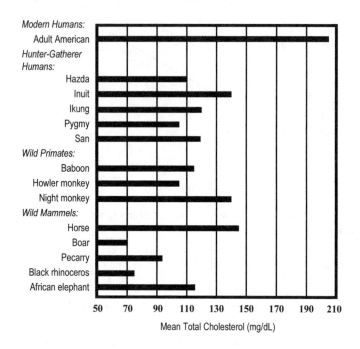

Figure 7.2. Total Cholesterol Levels in Various Populations

Total cholesterol levels for hunter-gatherers, wild primates, and wild mammals generally range from 70-140 mg/dL (LDL-C 35-70 mg/dL). In modern Westernized humans, mean total cholesterol levels (208 mg/dL; LDL-C 130 mg/dL) are almost twice these normal values, and atherosclerosis is present in up to 50% of individuals by age 50 (Arterioscler Thromb Vasc Biol 2002;22:849-54). In contrast, evidence from hunter-gatherer populations following the indigenous homosapien lifestyle indicate average total cholesterol levels of 100-150 mg/dL (LDL-C 50-75 mg/dL) and no evidence for atherosclerosis, even in individuals living into the eighth decade of life (Eur J Clin Nutr 2002;56:S42-52).

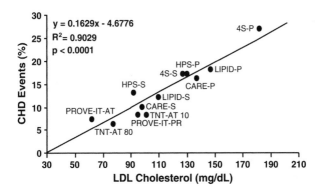

Figure 7.3. Relationship Between LDL Cholesterol and CHD Event Rates in Primary Prevention Trials

CHD event rates in primary prevention trials (4-5 years' duration) are directly proportional to LDL-C levels. P = placebo, S = statin. From: J Am Coll Cardiol 2004;43:2142-6.

2. **Statin vs. Statin Trials.** The most direct evidence to support the "lower-is-better" hypothesis comes from the Pravastatin or Atorvastatin Evaluation and Infection Trial (PROVE IT) (N Engl J Med 2004;350:495-504), the Treating to New Targets (TNT) trial (N Engl J Med 2005;352:1425-35), and the Incremental Decrease in Endpoints through Aggressive Lipid lowering (IDEAL) trial (JAMA 2005;294:2437-45). In these trials, intensive lowering of LDL-C resulted in significantly better cardiovascular outcomes (11%-22% reductions in major coronary events) compared to less intensive therapy.

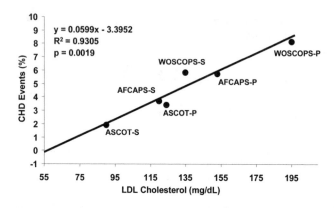

Figure 7.4. Relationship Between LDL Cholesterol and CHD Event Rates in Secondary Prevention Trials

CHD event rates in secondary prevention trials (5 years' duration except PROVE IT [2 years]) are directly proportional to LDL-C levels. AT = atorvastatin, AT 10 = atorvastatin 10 mg, AT 80 = atorvastatin 80 mg, P = placebo, PR = pravastatin, S = statin. Adapted from: J Am Coll Cardiol 2004;43:2142-6.

3. **Atherosclerosis Imaging Trials.** In the Reversal of Atherosclerosis with Aggressive Lipid Lowering (REVERSAL) trial, pravastatin 40 mg/d (on-treatment LDL-C 110 mg/dL) led to progression of atherosclerosis, whereas more intensive LDL-C lowering using atorvastatin 80 mg/d halted atherosclerosis progression (JAMA 2004;291:1132-34). Similar results using carotid intima-media thickness as an endpoint were obtained in the Atorvastatin vs. Simvastatin Atherosclerosis Progression (ASAP) trial (Lancet 2001;357:577-81) and in the Arterial Biology for the Investigation of the Treatment Effects of Reducing Cholesterol (ARBITER) trial (Circulation 2002;106:2055-60). And in A Study to Evaluate the Effect of Rosuvastatin on Intravascular Ultrasound-Derived Coronary Atheroma Burden (ASTEROID), intensive LDL-C lowering with rosuvastatin 40 mg/d (on-treatment LDL-C was 61 mg/dL) led to a significant regression of atherosclerosis (JAMA 2006;295:1556-65).

The ENHANCE study was a trial of 710 patients with familial hypercholesterolemia who were randomized to either simvastatin 80 mg/d or simvastatin 80 mg/d plus ezetimibe 10 mg/d. The carotid intima thickness, which was normal at baseline, progressed only minimally over the ensuing 2 years in both groups, without any statistically significant difference (N Engl J Med 2008;358:1431-43).

C.   Dyslipidemia Trials in Type 2 Diabetes

   1.   Statin Trials in Type 2 Diabetes. Four recent statin trials provide strong support for intensive LDL-C lowering in patients with type 2 diabetes: CARDS, ASCOT, HPS, and TNT. In <u>CARDS</u>, 2838 patients with type 2 diabetes, no clinical cardiovascular disease (absence of coronary, cerebrovascular, or severe peripheral vascular disease), LDL-C ≤ 160 mg/dL, and at least 1 other risk factor (hypertension, retinopathy, microalbuminuria, macroalbuminuria, current smoking) were randomized to atorvastatin 10 mg/d or placebo. (LDL-C was 119 mg/dL at baseline and 73 mg/dL on atorvastatin treatment.) At 4 years, atorvastatin reduced the first occurrence of any major vascular event by 37% (5.8% vs. 9.0%, p = 0.001) (Table 7.1). There was also a 27% reduction in all-cause mortality (borderline statistical significance). The absolute reduction in vascular events was 3.7%, and the number needed to treat x 4 years to prevent one major vascular event was only 27. It was estimated that 4 years of atorvastatin therapy in 1000 CARDS patients would prevent 37 first major cardiovascular events and 50 first or subsequent events. Benefits were consistent regardless of baseline lipid levels, gender, or age. Atorvastatin was also very well tolerated: there were no cases of rhabdomyolysis and no differences in muscle or liver adverse effects compared to placebo (Lancet 2004;364:685-96). In the diabetes substudy of <u>ASCOT</u>, 2553 type 2 diabetic patients (of 10,305 total patients) with well-controlled hypertension, no CHD, and average cholesterol levels were randomized to atorvastatin 10 mg/d or placebo. At 3.3 years, atorvastatin reduced major cardiovascular events or procedures by 23% (9.2% vs. 11.9%, p = 0.036) (Diabetes Care 2005;28:1151-7). Further positive results were demonstrated in the diabetes substudy of <u>HPS</u>, in which 5963 type 2 diabetic subjects (of 20,536 total patients in HPS) were randomized to simvastatin 40 mg/d or placebo. At 5 years, simvastatin reduced the first occurrence of any major vascular event (MI, coronary death, stroke, revascularization) by 22% (20.2% vs. 25.1% for placebo, p < 0.0001). There were also highly significant reductions among the 2912 diabetic subjects without occlusive arterial disease at entry (risk reduction 33%, p = 0.0003) and among the 2426 subjects with pretreatment LDL-C < 116 mg/dL (risk reduction 27%, p = 0.0007) (Lancet 2003;361:2005-16) (Table 7.2). It was estimated that 5 years of simvastatin would prevent 80 major vascular events per 1000 diabetic patients. In a post hoc analysis of 1501 diabetic patients with stable coronary heart disease in the TNT study, high-dose (80 mg/d) atorvastatin reduced major cardiovascular events by 25% at 4.9 years compared to atorvastatin 10 mg/d (Table 7.3).

2. **Fibrate Trials in Type 2 Diabetes.** Fibrates improve the lipid profile in diabetic dyslipidemia by lowering triglycerides by 20-50%, raising HDL-C by 5-20%, and shifting small, dense LDL-C particles to larger, less atherogenic particles. In the Fenofibrate Intervention and Event Lowering in Diabetes (FIELD) study, 9795 patients with type 2 diabetes (including 2131 with previous cardiovascular disease), total cholesterol of 115-250 mg/dL, total cholesterol/HDL-C ratio ≥ 4, and triglycerides of 90-445 mg/dL who were not on statin therapy at baseline were randomized to receive micronized fenofibrate 200 mg/d or placebo. At 1 year, LDL-C was reduced by 12%, HDL-C was increased by 4.5%, and triglycerides were reduced by 30% with fenofibrate compared with placebo. At 5 years, the primary endpoint of coronary events (CHD death or nonfatal MI) was not significantly different between treatment groups (hazard ratio 0.89, 95% CI 0.75-1.05; p = 0.16), but nonfatal MI was reduced by 24% (p = 0.01), coronary revascularization was reduced by 21% (p = 0.003), and total cardiovascular events were reduced by 11% (p = 0.035); microvascular disease, in particular retinopathy, was also reduced (Lancet 2005;366:1849-61). There were no significant reductions in CHD mortality (1.19 [95% CI 0.90–1.57]) or total mortality (1.11 [0.95–1.29]). These results are difficult to apply to clinical practice, however, because FIELD patients were not on statin therapy, as would be expected in clinical practice, and during the trial 17% of placebo patients and 8% of fenofibrate patients began other lipid-

lowering therapy, predominantly statins. Also, by the end of the study, HDL-C had only increased by 1%.

Major fibrate trials in study groups comprised of both diabetic and nondiabetic subjects include the Helsinki Heart Study, the Veterans Affairs HDL Intervention Trial (VA-HIT), and the Bezafibrate Infarction Prevention (BIP) study. In the <u>Helsinki Heart Study</u>, 4081 hypercholesterolemic middle-aged males without CHD were randomized to gemfibrozil or placebo. Gemfibrozil was associated with a 34% reduction in cardiac events without any significant reduction in total mortality (N Engl J Med 1987;317:1237-45). In <u>VA-HIT</u>, 2531 males with CHD, HDL cholesterol ≤ 40 mg/dL, and LDL cholesterol ≤ 140 mg/dL were randomized to gemfibrozil (1200 mg/d) or placebo. At 5 years, gemfibrozil decreased the risk for nonfatal MI or death from coronary causes by 22% (p = 0.006) without a significant reduction in total mortality (N Engl J Med 1999;341:410-8). In contrast, benefit was not demonstrated for bezafibrate at 6.2 years in the <u>BIP study</u>, except in patients with triglycerides ≥ 200 mg/dL at baseline (Circulation 2000;102:21, Circulation 2004;109:2197). Additional information is expected from the Action to Control Cardiovascular Risk in Diabetes (ACCORD) trial, in which approximately 10,000 patients with type 2 diabetes will receive both a fibrate and a statin to examine the effects of combined lowering of LDL-C and triglyceride and raising HDL-C on MI, stroke, and CHD death.

D. Therapeutic Implications. All patients with type 2 diabetes at increased risk for cardiovascular disease should receive statin therapy to reduce LDL-C by a *minimum of 30-40%*, regardless of baseline LDL-C levels. For diabetic patients *without* atherosclerotic vascular disease, NCEP ATP III guidelines recommend a minimum LDL-C target < 100 mg/dL (Circulation 2004;110:227-239). For diabetic patients *with* CHD or other clinical forms of atherosclerosis, the AHA/ACC secondary prevention guidelines state that it is reasonable to treat such patients to an LDL-C < 70 mg/dL (Circulation 2006;113:2363-2372). Use of minimal drug therapy to produce small changes in LDL-C to barely attain LDL-C goal is not recommended. Adjunctive pharmacotherapy is recommended for

Table 7.1. 4-Year Results of the Collaborative Atorvastatin Diabetes Study (CARDS)

	Atorvastatin 10 mg/d (n = 1428)	Placebo (n = 1410)	Relative Risk Reduction
Major vascular events* (%)	5.8	9.0	37%[†]
Acute coronary events (%)	3.6	5.5	36%
Coronary revascularization (%)	1.7	2.4	31%
Stroke (%)	1.5	2.8	48%

* Acute coronary heart disease death, nonfatal MI, hospitalized unstable angina, resuscitated cardiac arrest, coronary revascularization, stroke
† p = 0.001
From: Lancet 2004;364:685-96

Table 7.2. 5-Year Results of the Diabetes Substudy of the Heart Protection Study (HPS)

	Simvastatin 40 mg/d (n = 2978)	Placebo (n = 2985)	p-Value
Major coronary events (%)	9.4	12.6	< 0.0001
Nonfatal MI (%)	3.5	5.5	0.0002
Coronary death (%)	6.5	8.0	0.02
Stroke (%)	5.0	6.5	0.01
Revascularization (%)	8.7	10.4	0.02
Major vascular events* (%)	20.2	25.1	< 0.0001

* Nonfatal MI, coronary death, stroke, or revascularization procedure
From: Lancet 2003;361:2005-16

patients who remain above target LDL-C despite statins. Although studies generally did not include people < 40 years of age, it may be prudent to consider statin therapy in patients with diabetes under the age of 40 if they would have otherwise met criteria for these studies.

Table 7.3. 5-Year Results of the Treat to New Targets (TNT) Study in Diabetics: Post-hoc Analysis

	Atorvastatin 80 mg/d (n = 748)	Atorvastatin 10 mg/d (n = 753)	p-Value
Major cardiovascular events* (%)	13.8	17.9	0.026
Major cerebrovascular events (%)	7.0	10.0	0.037

* Death from CHD, nonfatal MI, resuscitated cardiac arrest, or fatal/nonfatal stroke.
From: N Engl J Med 2005;352:1425-35; American Diabetes Association Meeting, June, 2005, San Diego, CA

Goals of Therapy

LDL-C lowering is the primary goal of therapy for patients with type 2 diabetes. Non-HDL-C (LDL-C + VLDL-C), calculated by subtracting HDL-C from total cholesterol, is a secondary goal of therapy after LDL-C lowering in persons with triglycerides ≥ 200 mg/dL. LDL-C, non-HDL-C, and apo B goals in type 2 diabetic patients are < 100 mg/dL, < 130 mg/dL and < 90 mg/dL, respectively; targets < 70 mg/dL, < 100 mg/dL, and < 80 mg/dL are recommended for type 2 diabetic patients with CHD, other clinical forms of atherosclerosis, or ≥ 1 additional major cardiovascular risk factor (ADA/ACC Consensus Conference, J Am Coll Cardiol 2008;51:1512-24).

Treatment of Elevated LDL-C

The risk of cardiovascular events in type 2 diabetic subjects without known CHD is the same as the risk in nondiabetic subjects who have had a prior MI (Table 6.2, p. 96), and approximately 80% of diabetic individuals eventually die of a cardiovascular cause. Given the heightened risk of cardiovascular disease conferred by diabetes (risk of MI is 36% over 10 years), the National Cholesterol Education Program Adult Treatment Panel (ATP) III elevated diabetes to a "CHD risk equivalent" and recommended the same LDL-C targets and drug initiation levels for diabetic patients as for individuals with

CHD. Based on the results of HPS and other trials, an update from ATP III recommended that all patients with type 2 diabetes at increased risk of cardiovascular disease receive statin therapy to reduce LDL-C by *at least 30-40%* (Table 7.4) (Circulation 2004;110:227-239). More recently, based on two trials published subsequent to the ATP III update that further support the cardiovascular benefit for intensive LDL lowering — TNT and IDEAL (p. 113) — the AHA/ACC issued a 2006 update to their secondary prevention guidelines stating that it is reasonable to treat patients with CHD or other clinical forms of atherosclerotic disease to an LDL cholesterol < 70 mg/dL (Circulation 2006;113:2363-2372). Use of minimal drug therapy to produce small reductions in LDL-C to barely attain LDL-C goal is not recommended. If LDL-C levels at 6 weeks remain above target, intensification of diet and drugs, including add-on drug therapy, is recommended (Figure 7.5). Difficult-to-control patients should be referred to a lipid specialist.

Table 7.4. Doses of Statins Required to Attain an Approximate 30-40% Reduction in LDL-C Levels (Standard Doses)*

Drug	Dose (mg/d)	LDL-C Reduction (%)
Rosuvastatin	5-10	39-45
Atorvastatin	10	39
Simvastatin	20-40	35-41
Pravastatin	40	34
Lovastatin	40	31
Fluvastatin	40-80	25-35

Estimated LDL-C reductions were obtained from US Food and Drug Administration package inserts for each drug. For every doubling of the dose above the standard dose, an approximate 6% decrease in LDL-C levels can be obtained. Rosuvastatin is available in doses up to 40 mg; atorvastatin, simvastatin, pravastatin, lovastatin and fluvastatin are available in doses up to 80 mg. From: NCEP ATP III guideline update (Circulation 2004;110:227-239).

* Diabetic patients with established cardiovascular disease are at very high risk of cardiovascular events and frequently require ≥ 50% reductions in LDL-C levels to achieve an LDL-C target < 70 mg/dL (Table 7.5).

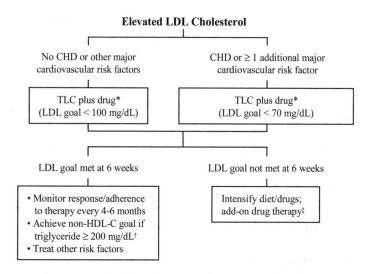

Figure 7.5. Treatment of Elevated LDL-C in Type 2 Diabetes

CHD = coronary heart disease; HDL-C= high-density lipoprotein; LDL-C = low-density lipoprotein; TLC = therapeutic lifestyle changes.

* Initial drug therapy usually consist of standard dose of a statin to reduce LDL-C levels by at least 30-40% (Table 7.4). For patients with CHD or other clinical forms of atherosclerosis, an LDL-C goal < 70 mg/dL is reasonable and frequently requires ≥ 50% reductions in LDL-C levels (Table 7.5). Use of minimal drug therapy to produce small reductions in LDL-C to barely attain LDL-C goal is not recommended.

† For triglyceride levels ≥ 200 mg/dL, non-HDL-C goal is < 130 mg/d. For patients with CHD or other clinical forms of atherosclerosis, a non-HDL-C goal < 100 mg/dL is reasonable. Non-HDL-C = total cholesterol minus HDL-C.

‡ If LDL-C levels at 6 weeks remain above LDL-C target, options include: (1) intensify diet therapy and consider adding plant sterols/stanols 2 gm/day and increasing soluble fiber to 10-25 gm/day; (2) intensify statin therapy; (3) add ezetimibe, a bile acid sequestrant, or niacin; (4) if elevated triglyceride or low HDL-C is present, consider adding niacin, a fibrate, or fish oil to statin therapy. Difficult-to-control patients should be referred to a lipid specialist.

Adapted from: NCEP ATP III update (Circulation 2004;110:227-239), AHA/ACC secondary prevention guideline update (Circulation 2006;113:2363-2372).

Table 7.5. Drug Doses Required to Attain ≥ 50% Reduction in LDL Cholesterol Levels

Drug	Dose (mg/d)	LDL Reduction (%)
Rosuvastatin	20*-40†	52-59
Atorvastatin	80†	51-54
Ezetimibe/simvastatin	10/20‡-10/80†	52-60

Estimated LDL-C reductions obtained from: Am J Cardiol 1998;81:582-7; Am J Cardiol 2003;92:152-60; Mayo Clin Proc 2004;79:620-9; Am Heart J 2004;148:e4.

* Optional starting dose

† Not recommended as starting dose per US Food and Drug Administration package inserts

‡ Recommended usual starting dose

Treatment of Low HDL-C and Elevated Triglyceride

A. **Low HDL-C.** HDL-C is involved in reverse cholesterol transport from the peripheral tissues to the liver. A depressed HDL-C level (< 40 mg/dL) is a powerful predictor of vascular risk. Causes of low HDL-C include elevated triglycerides, obesity, physical inactivity, cigarette smoking, high carbohydrate diets (> 60% of calories), type 2 diabetes, drugs (1st/2nd generation beta-blockers, anabolic steroids, progestational agents), and genetic factors. Nonpharmacologic measures that increase HDL-C include weight loss, exercise, smoking cessation, and low-glycemic diets that are high in monounsaturated fats, omega-3 fats, and lean protein. Alcohol raises HDL-C levels but is not recommended for that purpose. Once LDL-C and non-HDL-C goals are met, drug therapy to raise HDL-C may be considered for higher-risk individuals (Figure 7.6). ATP III does not establish a goal for HDL-C, but the American Heart Association recommends initiation of niacin or fibrate therapy in women with HDL-C < 50 mg/dL (Circulation 2004;109:672-93). The American Diabetes Association recommends an HDL-C level > 40 mg/dL (noting that an HDL-C > 50 mg/dL has been advocated in women), and suggests the use of a fibrate, niacin, or combination therapy with statin plus either fibrate or niacin to raise HDL-C levels (Diabetes

Care 2006;29:S4-42). It should be noted, however, that combination therapy with a statin plus a fibrate (especially gemfibrozil) increases the risk of muscle pain, elevated CPK levels, and rhabdomyolysis. TZDs and omega-3 fatty acids will each raise HDL-C levels in type 2 diabetes.

B. Elevated Triglyceride. Elevated triglyceride – especially postprandial hypertriglyceridemia (JAMA 2007;298:309-16) – is an independent risk factor for coronary disease. It is also associated with atherogenic VLDL-C remnants and small dense LDL-C particles, which correlate with the extent and progression of atherosclerosis. ATP III defines normal fasting triglyceride as < 150 mg/dL, borderline-high triglyceride as 150-199 mg/dL, high triglyceride as 200-499 mg/dL, and very high triglyceride as ≥ 500 mg/dL. Since remnant lipoproteins are comprised of partially degraded VLDL-C particles, elevated VLDL-C levels can be used as a marker for the presence of remnant lipoproteins and elevated risk. ATP III recognizes non-HDL-C (LDL-C + VLDL-C) as a secondary target of therapy in patients with high triglyceride (≥ 200 mg/dL) and sets the non-HDL-C goal at 30 mg/dL higher than the LDL-C goal (i.e., < 100 mg/dL in diabetics), based on the assumption that higher VLDL-C levels are associated with remnant lipoproteins and increased vascular risk. Non-HDL-C is determined by subtracting HDL-C from total cholesterol. Causes of elevated triglyceride include lifestyle-related causes (obesity, physical inactivity, cigarette smoking, excess alcohol intake, high carbohydrate diet), other secondary causes (diabetes mellitus, chronic renal failure, nephrotic syndrome, Cushing's disease, lipodystrophy, pregnancy, various drugs), and genetic causes. The potential benefits of lowering triglyceride levels are not as well studied as those of lowering LDL-C. For triglyceride levels of 150-199 mg/dL, emphasis is placed on therapeutic lifestyle changes, glycemic control, omega-3 fats, and LDL-C lowering; drug therapy to reduce triglycerides is not recommended (Figure 7.7). For triglyceride levels of 200-499 mg/dL, primary therapy is directed at LDL-C lowering, and non-HDL-C is a secondary goal of therapy. Drug therapy may be considered in high-risk patients to achieve the non-HDL-C goal. Pharmacologic approaches include intensification

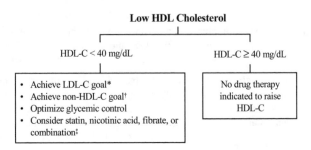

Figure 7.6. Treatment of Low HDL-C in Type 2 Diabetes

* LDL-C goal < 100 mg/dL; for patients with CHD or other clinical forms of atherosclerosis, it is reasonable to treat LDL-C to < 70 mg/dL (Circulation 2006;113:2363-2372). When indicated, drug therapy (statins preferred) should be used to reduce LDL-C by at least 30-40%.

† Non-HDL-C is a secondary goal of therapy after LDL-C lowering for persons with triglycerides ≥ 200 mg/dL. Non-HDL-C goal is < 130 mg/dL; for patients with CHD or other clinical forms of atherosclerosis, it is reasonable to treat non-HDL-C to < 100 mg/dL. Non-HDL-C = total cholesterol minus HDL-C.

‡ Monitor for worsening glycemic control (niacin) and for myopathy/rhabdomyolysis, especially with statin/fibrate or statin/niacin combination therapy. Fenofibrate has less risk of complications in combination therapy and is therefore the preferred fibrate.

of LDL-lowering therapy and/or the addition of high-dose omega-3 fatty acids (3-4 gm of EPA + DHA per day) or nicotinic acid or fibrates, when used with appropriate caution. For very high triglyceride levels (≥ 500 mg/dL), the primary goal of therapy is to prevent acute pancreatitis by rapidly lowering triglycerides to < 500 mg/dL with marked restriction of processed carbohydrates (i.e., avoidance of processed foods and drinks containing sugars or starches), weight reduction, increased physical activity, and the use of either a fibrate or nicotinic acid along with omega-3 fats. Once triglycerides are < 500 mg/dL, attention is directed toward achieving LDL-C and non-HDL-C targets.

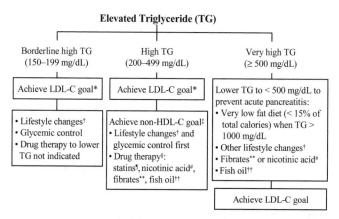

Figure 7.7. Treatment of Elevated Triglyceride in Type 2 Diabetes

*   LDL-C goal < 100 mg/dL; for patients with CHD or other clinical forms of atherosclerosis, it is reasonable to treat LDL-C to < 70 mg/dL. When indicated, drug therapy (statins preferred) should be used to lower LDL-C by at least 30-40%.

†   Weight control, increased physical activity, smoking cessation, restriction of alcohol in some, avoidance of high-carbohydrate diets (> 60% of total calories), discontinuation of nonessential drugs that raise cholesterol.

‡   Non-HDL-C goal < 130 mg/dL; for patients with CHD or other clinical forms of atherosclerosis, it is reasonable to treat non-HDL-C to < 100 mg/dL.

§   May need high-dose statin or moderate-dose statin plus either nicotinic acid or fibrate

¶   Statins lower triglycerides by 7-30% (20-50% or higher in patients with severely elevated triglyceride).

Nicotinic acid lowers triglycerides by 20-50%, but doses ≥ 2 gm/d can worsen hyperglycemia in persons with diabetes or insulin resistance.

** Fibrates lower triglycerides by 20-50% but can raise LDL-C in patients with hypertriglyceridemia. Fibrates are the best choice for acute reductions in triglycerides when used with appropriate caution.

†† Omega-3 fats (EPA + DHA) (3-4 gm/d) reduce triglycerides by 20-45% and are useful adjuncts to statin therapy. Lovaza , which contains highly purified omega-3 ethyl esters (EPA, DHA), has been approved by the FDA for the treatment of triglycerides ≥ 500 mg/dL; the dose in clinical studies was 4 gm/day.

Drug Therapy for Dyslipidemia

Drug therapy plays a central role in the management of dyslipidemia, improving lipid profile, slowing the progression of atherosclerosis, stabilizing rupture-prone plaques, reducing the risk of arterial thrombosis, and improving prognosis. For patients who require drug therapy, the drug should be added to, not substituted for, diet therapy and lifestyle modification. Table 7.6 lists effective cholesterol-lowering drugs.

A. **Statin Therapy.** Statins are overwhelmingly the drug class of choice for improving dyslipidemia and cardiovascular prognosis in type 2 diabetes. In addition to lowering LDL-C levels by 18-55%, statins lower the number of small, dense LDL-C particles, raise HDL-C levels by 5-10%, and lower triglycerides by 7-30%. The recent update to the National Cholesterol Education Program Adult Treatment Panel (ATP) III recommends that all type 2 diabetic patients at increased risk for cardiovascular disease should receive statin therapy to reduce LDL-C by *at least 30-40%*, regardless of baseline LDL-C levels (Table 7.4). A minimum LDL-C target < 100 mg/dL is recommended (Circulation 2004;110:227-239). Similar recommendations were published in guidelines from the American College of Physicians (ACP), which recommended that all type 2 diabetic patients should be treated with a statin regardless of LDL-C levels (Ann Intern Med 2004;140:644-9). Lower calculated LDL-C levels may be misleading in diabetes since LDL-C particles are often small but increased in number (and highly atherogenic); apoB or non-HDL cholesterol are better guides to the number of LDL-C particles in patients with type 2 diabetes. Based on two trials published subsequent to the ATP III update that further support the cardiovascular benefit of intensive LDL lowering — TNT and IDEAL (p. 113) — the AHA/ACC issued an update to their secondary prevention guidelines stating that it is reasonable to treat diabetic patients with CHD or other clinical forms of atherosclerotic disease to an LDL-C < 70 mg/dL (Circulation 2006;113:2363-2372). The role of statin therapy in lower-risk patients with type 2 diabetes (e.g., younger patients with LDL-C < 130 mg/dL and no other cardiovascular risk factors) awaits definition. (See Table 7.6 for contraindications and adverse effects.)

B. Adjuncts to Statin Therapy. Statin monotherapy may not achieve LDL-C goal or completely normalize the lipid profile in type 2 diabetes, and adjunctive pharmacotherapy may be required.

1. **Ezetimibe.** Ezetimibe inhibits the absorption of cholesterol and phytosterols from the small intestine. When used as monotherapy, ezetimibe lowers LDL-C by 18%. When added to statin therapy, ezetimibe 10 mg/d further reduces LDL-C by 23-25%, triglycerides by 10-15% and C-reactive protein by 10-20%, and raises HDL-C levels (Circulation 2003;107:2409-15, J Am Coll Cardiol 2002;40:2125-34, Am J Cardiol 2002;90:1084-91). (By comparison, each doubling of statin dose provides about 6% additional LDL-C reduction.) The combination of ezetimibe and statin is safe, effective and well tolerated, and is particularly helpful in the many diabetic patients who require ≥ 50% reductions in LDL-C levels. Ezetimibe in combination with simvastatin is available as a single tablet (Vytorin) in doses of 10/10 mg, 10/20 mg, 10/40 mg, and 10/80 mg. However, to date, no study is available to document that ezetimibe reduces either cardiovascular events or atherosclerotic progression.

2. **Niacin.** Niacin will raise HDL-C by 15-35% and lower LDL-C by 10-25%, triglycerides by 20-50%, and lipoprotein(a) by 20-30%. Niacin also improves prothrombotic tendencies by reducing plasminogen activator inhibitor-1 (PAI-1), fibrinogen, and alpha-2 antiplasmin levels. Niacin (and fibrates) can shift small, dense LDL-C particles toward larger, more buoyant particles, which may be less atherogenic. However, niacin can worsen insulin resistance, impair glucose tolerance, and raise HbA_{1c} levels in some diabetics, and there is an increased risk of myopathy/rhabdomyolysis when niacin is used, particularly at higher doses, in conjunction with a statin. When niacin is administered, lower doses (e.g., Niaspan < 1.5 gm/d) and glucose monitoring are recommended. Flushing can be decreased/prevented by taking aspirin 30-60 minutes prior to the dose. A novel niacin combination tablet is in development that holds promise to be a true "flush-free" niacin preparation. Niaspan in combination with simvastatin is available as a single tablet (Simcor).

3. **Omega-3 fatty acids.** Omega-3 fats, usually in the form of concentrated fish oil, are useful for diabetic dyslipidemia. Low doses

(1-1.5 gm/d) have been shown to reduce cardiovascular mortality, primarily by reducing sudden death; higher doses (3-4 gm/d) can lower triglycerides by 20-50% and are well-tolerated adjuncts to statins. The triglyceride-lowering effects of omega-3 fatty acids are additive to those noted with statin therapy. Lovaza, formerly Omacor, contains highly purified omega-3 ethyl esters (85% EPA + DHA) and is approved for the treatment of triglycerides $\geq$ 500 mg/dL; the dose in clinical studies was 4 gm/day.

4.   **Fibrates.** Fibrates improve the lipid profile in diabetic dyslipidemia by lowering triglycerides by 20-50%, raising HDL-C by 16-35%, and shifting small, dense LDL-C particles to larger, less atherogenic particles. However, the risk for myopathy and rhabdomyolysis is increased when fibrates are used with statins, with the possible exception of fenofibrate (Drug Metab Dispos 2002;30:1280-7).

5.   **Bile acid sequestrants.** These drugs act by irreversibly binding bile acid salts in the gut, with subsequent excretion in the stool. Because bile acids are synthesized from cholesterol in the liver, bile acid sequestrants lower blood cholesterol levels. When administered according to dosing guidelines, bile acid sequestrants typically reduce LDL cholesterol by 15-30%. HDL cholesterol may increase slightly (by 3-5%), and plasma triglycerides are usually not affected but may increase. LDL-lowering effects may occur as early as 4-7 days, and maximum effects are usually evident within 1 month. First-generation bile acid sequestrants (cholestyramine and colestipol) are poorly tolerated due to GI side effects (especially constipation) and interference with the absorption of many drugs. Colesevelam is a newer, more convenient (3 pills twice daily), well-tolerated bile acid sequestrant that does not interfere with the absorption of other drugs. In addition to its cholesterol-lowering effects, colesevelam is now approved to lower blood glucose as well, and typically reduces HbA1c by 0.5%.

Table 7.6. Effective Lipid-Modifying Drug Therapy

Drug (usual starting/max dose)	Lipid Effects	Comments
HMG-CoA Reductase Inhibitors (Statins)		
Atorvastatin (10/80 mg/d) Fluvastatin (40/80 mg/d) Lovastatin (20/80 mg/d) Pravastatin (20/80 mg/d) Rosuvastatin (5/40 mg/d) Simvastatin (20/80 mg/d)	LDL-C: ↓ 18-55% HDL-C: ↑ 5-15% TG: ↓ 7-30%	*Major use:* Overwhelmingly the drug class of choice for elevated LDL-C levels. Highly effective for lowering LDL-C and preventing cardiovascular and cerebrovascular events. *Absolute CI:* active or chronic liver disease, pregnancy, lactation. *Relative CI:* concomitant use of cyclosporine, macrolide antibiotics, various antifungal drugs, cytochrome P-450 inhibitors; previous intolerance to statins due to myalgias, elevated liver transaminases, other side effects. *Adverse effects:* myopathy, ↑ liver transaminases. Fibrates and nicotinic acid should be used with caution in combination with statins.
Cholesterol Absorption Inhibitor		
Ezetimibe (10 mg/d)	LDL-C: ↓ 18 (as monotherapy); further ↓ by 25% when added to statins HDL-C: ↑ 1% TG: ↓ 8%	*Major use:* Safe, effective, and well-tolerated adjunct to statins when further LDL-C lowering is required. Not recommended in moderate or severe hepatic insufficiency. Effectiveness reduced when given within 2-4 hours of bile acid sequestrant. *CI:* combination with statin in patients with active liver disease or unexplained persistent transaminase elevations. *Adverse effects:* GI complaints.

↑ = increases, ↓ = decreases, CI = contraindication, HDL-C= HDL cholesterol, LDL = LDL cholesterol, Lp(a) = lipoprotein(a), TG = triglyceride

Table 7.6. Effective Lipid-Modifying Drug Therapy

Drug (usual starting/max dose)	Lipid Effects	Comments
Nicotinic Acid (Niacin)		
Immediate-release form (50 mg/4.5 gm/d) Sustained-release form (500 mg/2 gm/d) Extended-release form (500 mg/2 gm/d)	LDL-C: ↓ 5-25% HDL-C: ↑ 15-35% TG: ↓ 20-50%	*Major use:* Useful in nearly all dyslipidemias. Uniquely effective in atherogenic dyslipidemia. Also useful for elevated Lp(a) levels and as adjunctive therapy for mixed dyslipidemia. *Absolute CI:* chronic liver disease, severe gout. *Relative CI:* hyperuricemia, high doses (> 3 gm/d) in type 2 diabetes. Caution in active liver or peptic ulcer disease, hyperuricemia, gout. *Adverse effects:* flushing, hyperglycemia, hyperuricemia/gout, upper GI distress, hepatotoxicity (esp. sustained-release).
Bile Acid Sequestrants		
Colesevelam (3.8/4.4 gm/d) Cholestyramine ([4-16]/24 gm/d) Colestipol ([5-20]/30 gm/d)	LDL-C: ↓ 15-20% HDL-C: ↑ 3-5% TG: usually not affected; may ↑	*Major use:* Colesevelam recently FDA-approved for lowering blood glucose; other resins have similar effects (lower HbA1c by ~ 0.5%). Moderate hypercholesterolemia, younger patients with elevated LDL-C, and women with elevated LDL-C who are considering pregnancy (sequestrants are not absorbed out of the GI tract and lack systemic toxicity). Also useful as adjunctive therapy with statins. *Absolute CI:* familial dysbetalipoproteinemia, triglyceride > 400 mg/dL. *Relative CI:* triglyceride > 200 mg/dL. *Adverse effects:* GI complaints common, decreased absorption of several drugs.

Table 7.6. Effective Lipid-Modifying Drug Therapy

Drug (usual starting/max dose)	Lipid Effects	Comments
Fibric Acid Derivatives		
Gemfibrozil (600 mg bid) Fenofibrate (130-200 mg/d) Clofibrate (1000 mg bid)	LDL-C: ↓ 5-20% (may ↑ LDL-C if ↑ TG at baseline) HDL-C: ↑ 10-35% TG: ↓ 20-50%	*Major uses:* Hypertriglyceridemia, atherogenic dyslipidemia (especially in type 2 diabetes). *Absolute CI:* severe hepatic or renal dysfunction, primary biliary cirrhosis, gallbladder disease. *Relative CI:* combined therapy with statins (occasional occurrence of severe myopathy or rhabdomyolysis). Use with caution when combining with coumarin anticoagulants or cyclosporine. *Adverse effects:* dyspepsia, upper GI complaints, cholesterol gallstones, myopathy, multiple drug-drug interactions with gemfibrozil.
Omega-3 Fatty Acids (Fish Oil)		
Omega-3 acid ethyl esters (4 gm/d)	TG: ↓ 45% non-HDL-C: ↓ 14% LDL-C: ↑ 44% HDL-C: ↑ 9%	*Major use:* Hypertriglyceridemia (TG ≥500 mg/dL). *CI:* Use with caution in patients with known hypersensitivity or allergy to fish, and in women who are pregnant or breastfeeding. *Adverse effects:* eructation, dyspepsia, taste perversion.

↑ = increases, ↓ = decreases, CI = contraindication, HDL-C= HDL cholesterol, LDL-C = LDL cholesterol, Lp(a) = lipoprotein(a), TG = triglyceride

Chapter 8

Control of Hypertension in Type 2 Diabetes

Hypertension affects 50 million Americans and 1 billion individuals worldwide, including approximately 3 out of 4 persons with type 2 diabetes. Twelve percent of Americans have both diabetes and hypertension (Am J Prev Med 2002;22:42-48, J Am Geriatr Soc 2001;49:109–16, Diabetes Care 1998;21:1414–31). The prevalence of hypertension is 2-fold higher and the incidence of cardiovascular events is 6-fold higher in diabetic patients compared to nondiabetic age-matched subjects (Diabetes Care 2005;28:Suppl 1, Arch Intern Med 1989;149:1942–5, JAMA 1967;202:104–10). Numerous epidemiological and observational studies demonstrate a direct, continuous relationship between increasing blood pressure and vascular risk, with no apparent lower threshold (although data are lacking below a blood pressure of 115/75 mmHg) (Lancet 2002;360:1903-1913, J Hypertens 2000;18:1193-1196). Systolic, diastolic, mean arterial, and pulse pressures all predict vascular risk, although systolic and diastolic blood pressures are recommended as the best means of classifying blood pressure (Circulation 2005;111:697-716). Among individuals aged 55-65 years without hypertension at baseline, the residual lifetime risk of developing hypertension is 90% (JAMA 2002;287:1003-10).

More than 90-95% of hypertension is idiopathic (essential), while 5-10% can be ascribed to an identifiable cause (secondary hypertension). Essential hypertension is caused by increased vascular reactivity and/or inappropriate renal retention of salt and water. Diabetic subjects are especially prone to these problems due to a hyperactive renin-angiotensin-aldosterone system and increased sympathetic tone. In addition, hyperglycemia increases salt and water retention since, for every molecule of glucose filtered and reabsorbed in the kidney, one molecule of sodium is also absorbed. Over many years, this leads to accelerated atherosclerosis in large vessels, obliterative changes and/or thinning and rupture of small vessels, and increased workload on the heart. Intensive treatment of hypertension in diabetic patients reduces by 30% the incidence of and fatality from coronary heart disease, stroke, heart failure, and kidney disease. Blood pressure control also reduces the progression of diabetic retinopathy and deterioration in visual acuity (BMJ 1998;317:703-13).

Hypertension is grossly underdiagnosed and undertreated. Results from the Third National Health and Nutrition Evaluation Survey (NHANES III) indicated that 29% of diabetic individuals with hypertension were unaware of the diagnosis; 43% of diabetic individuals with hypertension were untreated; 55% of treated diabetic individuals had a blood pressure ≥ 140/90 mmHg; and only 12% of treated diabetic individuals had a blood pressure < 130/85 mmHg (Am J Rev Med 2002;22:42-48). Using NHANES III data, it was estimated that proper control of hypertension could prevent 19-56% and 31-57% of coronary events in men and women, respectively (Am Heart 2003;145:888-895).

Diagnosis of Hypertension

Blood pressure targets for diabetic patients are lower than for the general population. Hypertension in a diabetic patient is defined by a systolic BP ≥ 130 mmHg or a diastolic BP ≥ 80 mmHg, based on the average of two or more readings at two or more visits after the initial screen. (In JNC 7, for the general population, hypertension is defined by a BP ≥ 140/90 mmHg.) A single recording may be sufficient if systolic blood pressure is ≥ 210 mmHg or diastolic blood pressure is ≥ 120 mmHg, especially if symptoms are present, but even very high elevations in blood pressure may occur transiently during extreme stress or acute illness.

Treatment of Diabetic Hypertension

A. **Overview.** Cardiovascular events are 2-4–fold higher in diabetic hypertensives compared to nondiabetic hypertensives, and aggressive blood pressure lowering is recommended in all diabetic subjects to reduce the risk of cardiovascular events, retinopathy, and nephropathy. In the United Kingdom Diabetes Prevention Study (UKPDS) epidemiological study, each 10-mmHg reduction in mean systolic BP decreased the risk of diabetes-related death by 15%, MI by 11%, and microvascular complications by 13% (BMJ 1998;317:703-13). In the Hypertension Optimum Treatment (HOT) study, there was a 51% reduction in cardiovascular events for diabetic patients assigned to a diastolic BP target of 80 mmHg versus a target of 90 mmHg in spite of only a 4 mmHg difference in systolic BP (Lancet 1998;351: 1755-62). Based on these and other data, the Seventh Report of the Joint National Committee on Prevention, Detection, Evaluation, and Treatment of High Blood Pressure (JNC 7) recommends a target BP level of < 130/80 mmHg in patients with type 2 diabetes (JAMA 2003;289:2560-72). This goal has been endorsed by the ADA and the AACE/ACE. The National Kidney Foundation has set a BP goal ≤ 125/75 mmHg for individuals with diabetic nephropathy (i.e., the presence of ≥ 1 gm of protein in a 24-hour urine specimen). Treating to BP ≤ 120/75 mmHg may be even more effective at halting the progression of renal disease and vascular complications, especially for persons with proteinuria > 1 gm/d (Endocr Pract 2006;12:193-222).

B. Blood Pressure Goals. In the setting of type 2 diabetes, the goal of therapy is to reduce BP to < 130/80 mmHg. Optimal BP is ≤ 120/75 mmHg. To achieve maximum benefit, systolic and diastolic BP should be reduced to established targets and, based on recent data, rapid lowering of BP is important to reduce MI and stroke (see next page). Despite marked benefits of antihypertensive therapy, only 12% of diabetic patients in the U.S. are well controlled (BP < 130/80 mmHg) (Am J Rev Med 2002;22:42-8).

C. Therapeutic Lifestyle Changes (Chapter 4). Therapeutic lifestyle changes should be initiated simultaneously with drug therapy for diabetic patients with systolic BP ≥ 130 mmHg. Measures advocated by JNC 7 include: weight control; limit alcohol to no more than 2 drinks/day (1 oz or 30 mL of ethanol [24 oz beer, 10 oz wine, or 3 oz 80-proof whiskey]) in most men and no more than 1 drink/day in women and lighter-weight persons; increase aerobic physical activity to 30-45 minutes most days of the week; reduce sodium intake to ≤ 100 mmol/d (2.4 gm/d sodium or 6 gm/d sodium chloride); maintain adequate intake of dietary potassium (approximately 90 mmol/d), calcium, magnesium; smoking cessation; and increase dietary intake of fruits, vegetables, and low-fat dairy and reduce intake of saturated fat and total fat.

D. Initial Drug Therapy. The average diabetic patient with hypertension requires 3.2 drugs to achieve/maintain target BP, with each antihypertensive agent lowering the systolic BP by approximately 10-15 mmHg. In the absence of contraindications, and based on the proven cardioprotective/renoprotective properties of ARBs and ACE inhibitors in diabetic patients, initial therapy with an ARB or ACE inhibitor in combination with a low-dose thiazide diuretic (e.g., hydrochlorothiazide 12.5 mg/d) is a reasonable approach (Figure 8.1). Recently, more effective blockade of the renin-angiotensin system (RAS) has become possible with the availability of the direct renin inhibitor aliskiren. For individuals with chronic renal insufficiency (GFR < 50 mL/min), a loop diuretic should be used instead of a thiazide diuretic. Addition of a diuretic will potentiate the antihypertensive effects of ARBs and ACE inhibitors and offset their tendency to induce hyperkalemia. If monotherapy is employed, an ARB or ACE inhibitor is recommended, followed, if necessary, by a thiazide diuretic. (Consider doubling the usual starting dose of an ACE inhibitor or ARB if the patient is African American.) A beta-blocker or a calcium antagonist may also be considered for second-line therapy, but these agents are commonly reserved for the more than 50% of diabetic patients who require additional drug therapy after an ARB (or ACE inhibitor) and diuretic. Recent hypertension guidelines from AACE identify a BP goal ≤ 130/80 for individuals with diabetes (≤ 120/75 mmHg for proteinuria ≥ 1 gm/d) and recommend an ARB or ACE inhibitor as a first- or second-line agent, a thiazide diuretic (at low-dose with potassium replacement or a potassium-sparing diuretic) as a first- or second-line agent, a beta blocker (preferably one with alpha-blockade, e.g., carvedilol) as a second- or third-line agent, and a calcium antagonist (preferably a nondihydropyridine) as a second-, third-, or fourth-line agent (Endocr Pract 2006;12:193-222). Once-daily, fixed-dose combination drug therapy (e.g., ARB or ACE in combination with a diuretic) may improve patient compliance by minimizing pill burden. Low-dose aspirin (81 mg/d), recommended for most type 2 diabetic patients, may further reduce blood pressure when administered before bedtime (J Am Coll Cardiol 2005;46:975-83). Each antihypertensive agent can be expected to lower the systolic blood pressure by about 10-15 mmHg. Patients

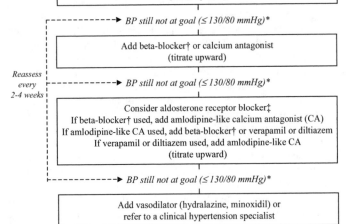

Blood Pressure (BP) > 130/80 mmHg*
(2 or more measurement at least 2 weeks apart)

Start ARB or ACE inhibitor plus thiazide diuretic‡
Consider monotherapy with ARB or ACE inhibitor for systolic BP
< 20 mmHg of goal (i.e., 131-150 mmHg); add diuretic as needed
(titrate upward)

*BP still not at goal (≤ 130/80 mmHg)**

Add beta-blocker† or calcium antagonist
(titrate upward)

*BP still not at goal (≤ 130/80 mmHg)**

Consider aldosterone receptor blocker‡
If beta-blocker† used, add amlodipine-like calcium antagonist (CA)
If amlodipine-like CA used, add beta-blocker† or verapamil or diltiazem
If verapamil or diltiazem used, add amlodipine-like CA
(titrate upward)

*BP still not at goal (≤ 130/80 mmHg)**

Add vasodilator (hydralazine, minoxidil) or
refer to a clinical hypertension specialist

Reassess every 2-4 weeks

Figure 8.1. Treatment of Diabetic Hypertension

ACE = angiotensin converting enzyme, ARB = angiotensin II receptor blocker.
* BP goal is ≤ 125/75 mmHg for nephropathy plus proteinuria > 1 gm/day.
  Treat systolic and diastolic BP to goal. Drug therapy should be initiated
  concurrently with smoking cessation, weight control, physical activity. Most
  diabetic patients require at least 2 drugs to control BP and many require 3 or
  more. Check for postural hypotension prior to adjustments in drug therapy.
  Home BP recordings are recommended to optimize therapy
† Based on GEMINI (p. 143), carvedilol substantially lowers BP when used with
  an ACE inhibitor and does not worsen insulin resistance or glycemic control
‡ For chronic renal insufficiency (GFR < 50 mL/min), substitute a loop diuretic
  (e.g., furosemide BID or torsemide QD) for a thiazide diuretic; only use
  aldosterone receptor blocker if K^+ < 4.8 mEq/L on ARB or ACE inhibitor

should be encouraged to record and report home blood pressure measurements to assess the effectiveness of antihypertensive drug therapy and to detect white-coat and reverse white-coat hypertension.

E. **Rapidity of Blood Pressure Lowering and Intensification of Drug Therapy.** Recent data indicate important cardiovascular benefits for rapid control of blood pressure. In VALUE, 15,245 high-risk hypertensive patients (32% with type 2 diabetes) were randomized to valsartan or amlodipine. Controlled BP at 6 months was associated with a 25% reduction in fatal and nonfatal cardiac events ($p < 0.05$), with benefits as early as 1 month for immediate responders (Lancet 2004;363:2049-51, Lancet 2004;363:2022-31). Therefore, if systolic BP remains ≥ 130 mmHg at 2 weeks after initial therapy, drug dosages should be optimized or drugs from different drug classes should be added at 3-4–week intervals. A beta-blocker, preferably one with alpha-1 blockade (e.g., carvedilol), which does not increase insulin resistance or worsen hyperglycemia, or a calcium antagonist (e.g., amlodipine, verapamil, diltiazem) is an excellent option for diabetic patients who require additional drug therapy to lower blood pressure after an ARB (or ACE inhibitor) and diuretic. An aldosterone receptor blocker (spironolactone, eplerenone) and/or a centrally-acting vasodilator (hydralazine, minoxidil) may be useful if further drug therapy is required; with an aldosterone receptor blocker, monitoring for hyperkalemia should be performed on days 3, 10, and 21 of therapy. Before proceeding to each successive treatment step, potential reasons for lack of responsiveness should be identified, including pseudohypertension, nonadherence to therapy, volume overload, drug-related causes, and secondary causes of hypertension such as hyperaldosteronism, which can be diagnosed with an elevated aldosterone-to-renin ratio and responds well to anti-aldosterone drugs such as spironolactone and eplerenone. Hospitalization should be considered for patients with BP $\geq 200/120$ mmHg and symptomatic target organ damage.

Use of Specific Drug Therapy

A. **ACE Inhibitors.** ACE inhibitors improve event-free survival in patients with atherosclerotic vascular disease, systolic heart failure, asymptomatic left ventricular (LV) dysfunction, or acute myocardial infarction (Circulation 2005;112:1339-1346, Lancet 2003;362:782–8, N Engl J Med 2000;342:145–53, Lancet 2000;355:1575–81, Circulation 1995;92:3132–7). They also exert renoprotective effects in type 1 diabetes and have been shown to reduce proteinuria and progression to overt nephropathy in type 2 diabetes (Lancet 2000;35:253–9), although a specific renoprotective effect beyond blood pressure lowering in pre-existing diabetic nephropathy has been questioned (Lancet 2005;366:2026-2033). A recent meta-analysis found that ACE inhibitors reduced the incidence of newly diagnosed type 2 diabetes by 27% (J Am Coll Cardiol 2005;46:821-6), although no drug has yet been approved for the prevention of diabetes. Antihypertensive effects usually become apparent within one week and are augmented by the addition of a low-dose thiazide diuretic (e.g., hydrochlorothiazide 12.5 mg) or a calcium channel blocker (e.g., amlodipine). In the Avoiding Cardiovascular Events in Combination Therapy in Patients Living with Hypertension (ACCOMPLISH) trial, 11,462 high-risk hypertensive patients (with heart disease, renal disease, or other target organ damage) were randomized to either benazepril plus hydrochlorothiazide (HCTZ) or to benazepril plus amlodipine. Sixty percent of patients had diabetes. At a mean follow-up of 39 months, therapy with benazepril/amlodipine reduced cardiovascular morbidity and mortality by 20%, compared to therapy with benazepril/HCTZ (presented at the American College of Cardiology meeting, March, 2008, Chicago, IL). Cough develops in 10%-20% of patients receiving ACE inhibitors and may require discontinuation of therapy. These patients can usually be switched to an ARB without recurrence of cough. Approximately 0.5% of patients (the percentage is higher in African Americans) receiving ACE inhibitors develop angioneurotic edema. ACE inhibitors should be immediately discontinued if symptoms develop, and switching to an ARB does not decrease the risk of this potentially life-threatening complication.

Diabetic patients receiving ACE inhibitors should not be treated routinely with potassium supplement or potassium-sparing diuretics, especially if renal insufficiency is present, due to the increased risk of hyperkalemia. Intravascular volume depletion should be corrected (e.g., withholding diuretics or increasing salt intake for several days) before initiating therapy to reduce the risk of symptomatic hypotension. ACE inhibitors should not be used during pregnancy (category D for second and third trimesters; category C for first trimester), and when pregnancy is detected, ACE inhibitors should be discontinued as soon as possible.

B. Angiotensin Receptor Blockers (ARBs). ARBs are effective antihypertensive agents with proven cardioprotective properties in patients with hypertensive LVH, heart failure, and acute MI (Lancet 2002;359;995-1003, Lancet 2003;362:772-6, N Engl J Med 2003;349:1893-906). They also exert cardioprotective effects in patients with vascular disease or high-risk diabetes (see ONTARGET trial, p. 155). In addition, ARBs exert renoprotective effects, reducing proteinuria and slowing the deterioration in renal function in diabetic nephropathy, as measured by occurrence of doubling of serum creatinine or end-stage renal disease (need for dialysis or renal transplantation)(N Engl J Med 2001;345:861-9, N Engl J Med 2001;345:851-60, N Engl J Med 2001;345:870-8), although a specific renoprotective effect beyond blood pressure lowering in patients with pre-existing diabetic nephropathy has been questioned (Lancet 2005;366:2026-2033). In the LIFE trial, losartan reduced the risk of the composite endpoint of death, MI, or stroke to a greater extent than atenolol in hypertensive patients with LVH (Lancet 2002;359;995-1003). A meta-analysis found that ARBs reduced the incidence of newly diagnosed type 2 diabetes by 23% (J Am Coll Cardiol 2005;46:821-6), although no drug has yet been approved for the prevention of diabetes. ARBs are very well tolerated, with an overall incidence of adverse effects similar to placebo. Antihypertensive effects usually become apparent within one week and are augmented by the addition of a low-dose thiazide diuretic (e.g., hydrochlorothiazide 12.5 mg) or a calcium channel blocker. Most patients who experience a persistent dry cough in response to an ACE inhibitor can be switched to an ARB without recurrence of cough. Diabetic patients receiving ARBs should not be treated routinely with potassium supplement or potassium-sparing diuretics, especially if renal insufficiency is present, due to the risk of hyperkalemia. Intravascular volume depletion should be corrected (e.g., withholding diuretics or increasing salt intake for several days) before initiating therapy to reduce the risk of symptomatic hypotension. Patients who experience angioneurotic edema with an ACE inhibitor are at high risk for this potentially life-threatening complication with ARBs. ARBs should not be used during pregnancy (category D for 2nd/3rd trimesters; category C for 1st trimester); when pregnancy is detected, ARBs should be discontinued.

C. **Renin Inhibitors.** Pharmacological inhibition of the renin-angiotensin system (RAS) via ACE inhibitors and ARBs have been proven to reduce morbidity and mortality in diabetic patients with hypertension, atherosclerosis, nephropathy, and heart failure. The direct renin inhibitor aliskiren has been developed as an alternative to ACE inhibitors and ARBs and a more complete means of blocking the RAS. In clinical studies, the addition of aliskiren to an ARB further reduced the risk of proteinuria among diabetic subjects by 19% (AVOID study), and the effect of aliskiren on blood pressure is additive when combined with an ARB, a thiazide diuretic, or a calcium channel blocker. No data on the use of aliskiren combined with a beta-blocker are available; however, since beta-blockers decrease renin release by 30-55%, combination therapy should be efficacious. In the Aliskiren Observation of Heart Failure Treatment (ALOFT) study, the addition of aliskiren to beta-blocker and ACE-inhibitor therapy resulted in a significant decrease in pro-BNP, indicating improvement in heart failure (presented at the European Society of Cardiology Congress meeting, September, 2007, Vienna, Austria; also available at theheart.org). In the Aliskiren Left Ventricular Assessment of Hypertrophy (ALLAY) study, aliskiren proved as effective in reducing left ventricular mass at 36 months in patients with hypertension as losartan (presented at the American College of Cardiology meeting, March, 2008, Chicago, IL; also available at the heart.org). There is a very low incidence of cough with aliskiren, but the risk of angioneurotic edema is still present. The drug should not be used in pregnancy and is associated with diarrhea and a slight increase in the frequency of gout and uric acid kidney stones. Aliskiren has been shown to be equally effective at lowering blood pressure in diabetic and nondiabetic patients (Pharmacokinet 2006;45:1125-34).

D. Diuretics. Diuretics are effective first-line agents in general population studies. However, when treating patients with diabetes they should be used as second-line therapy or as part of combination therapy with an ARB, an ACE inhibitor, or a direct renin inhibitor to potentiate blood pressure lowering. Low-dose hydrochlorothiazide in fixed-dose combination with an ARB or ACE inhibitor is often used as first-line therapy in diabetic patients. Recommended starting and maximal doses for diuretics are the equivalent of 12.5 mg and 25 mg of hydrochlorothiazide, respectively. Higher doses increase insulin resistance, worsen glycemic control, lower HDL cholesterol, and increase triglyceride and uric acid levels. In ALLHAT, use of chlorthalidone in doses equivalent to 50 mg hydrochlorothiazide resulted in 30% more individuals being diagnosed with diabetes compared to amlodipine or lisinopril (JAMA 2002;288:2981-97, JAMA 2000;283;1967-75). For individuals with chronic renal insufficiency (GFR < 50 mL/min), a loop diuretic should be used instead of a thiazide diuretic. The major antihypertensive response to diuretics is seen within 1-2 weeks of starting therapy or adjusting the dose. Patients with moderate renal insufficiency and volume-dependant hypertension who do not response to thiazides may require a loop diuretic (furosemide, bumetanide), a high-potency diuretic (metolazone, indapamide, or the longer-acting torsemide), or a combination of metolazone plus a loop diuretic. Potassium-sparing diuretics should generally be avoided in diabetic patients with renal insufficiency and in those receiving potassium supplements, ACE inhibitors, or ARBs. If triple therapy does not achieve the desired blood pressure goal, the patient should be screened for primary hyperaldosteronism with a plasma aldosterone (pg/dL)-to-renin ratio. In fact, all patients with a serum $K^+ < 4.0$ meq/L at baseline should probably be screened for hyperaldosteronism prior to initiating antihypertensive therapy. If this ratio exceeds 25-30, then more definitive investigations are required. If the diagnosis is confirmed, then spironolactone or eplerenone becomes the major form of therapy.

E. Beta Blockers. Type 2 diabetes disrupts normal autonomic balance, predisposing to excessive sympathetic tone and increasing the risk of hypertension, coronary disease, and sudden cardiac death. Diabetic patients have a 3-fold increased risk of sudden death compared to nondiabetic patients. First and second generation beta blockers may worsen insulin resistance, mask symptoms of hypoglycemia, and induce peripheral vasoconstriction, which can worsen peripheral arterial disease in the diabetic patient. Nevertheless, they are effective antihypertensive agents with proven benefits on survival following acute MI and in stable systolic heart failure. They also reduce cardiovascular events at least as well (and possibly better) in diabetic patients as they do in nondiabetic patients, including a 50% reduction in sudden death. Beta blockers are recommended for diabetic patients who require additional drug therapy to lower blood pressure after an ARB (or ACE inhibitor) and diuretic. Beta blockers with alpha-1 blockade, such as carvedilol, are particularly useful in diabetic patients: the 7% alpha-1 blockade is enough to lower insulin resistance, and the resulting difference in insulin sensitivity when carvedilol is compared with a 1st or 2nd generation beta blocker is equivalent to that seen with a thiazolidinedione. The improvement in insulin resistance seen with alpha-1 blockade is due to vasodilation of the vascular bed in muscle, which is an advantage to the diabetic patient. Since insulin resistance and hypertensive ventricular remodeling in type 2 diabetes start long before the development of heart failure, early use of beta blockers to reverse remodeling will benefit the diabetic patient. Among 3029 patients with chronic heart failure randomized to carvedilol or metoprolol in the COMET trial, carvedilol reduced all-cause mortality by 17% (34% vs. 40%, p = 0.0017) and new diabetes by 22% at 4.8 years (Lancet 2003;362:7-13). In GEMINI, 1235 patients with type 2 diabetes and hypertension receiving a renin-angiotensin-system blocker (ACE inhibitor or ARB) were randomized to carvedilol 6.25-25 mg twice daily or metoprolol 50-200 mg twice daily. At 35 weeks, carvedilol resulted in better glycemic control (HbA$_{1c}$ levels stabilized with carvedilol but increased with metoprolol), improved insulin sensitivity (insulin resistance was reduced by carvedilol but increased with metoprolol), and less progression to microalbuminuria (JAMA 2004;292:2227-36) (Table 8.1). Beta blockers with alpha-1 blockade are generally well tolerated; however, due to alpha-1 blockade, the risk of postural hypotension is increased, and concomitant use of phosphodiesterase inhibitors such as

Table 8.1. Results of the Glycemic Effects in Diabetes Mellitus: Carvedilol-Metoprolol Comparison in Hypertensives (GEMINI) Trial

Parameter (Results at 35 weeks)	Carvedilol (n = 454)	Metoprolol (n = 657)	p-Value
Mean change in HbA1c from baseline	0.02	0.15	0.004*
Insulin sensitivity	- 9.1	- 2.0	0.04†
Progression to microalbuminuria	6.6	11.1	0.03

* P-value for the mean difference between groups with respect to the change in HbA1c from baseline (primary outcome). HbA1c was stabilized with carvedilol but increased with metoprolol.

† Insulin resistance was reduced by carvedilol but increased with metoprolol.

From: JAMA 2004;292:2227-2236.

sildenafil (Viagra), tadalafil (Cialis), and vardenafil (Levitra) is not recommended. Nevibulol is a new beta blocker that combines a high degree of beta-1 selectivity with endothelium-dependent vasodilating effects that has been shown to lower blood pressure in patients with mild to moderate hypertension and is well tolerated (J Clin Hypertens 2007;9:667-676). Beta blockers should not be given to patients with marked sinus bradycardia, greater than first-degree AV block or sick sinus syndrome without a functioning pacemaker, or severe decompensated heart failure, and they should be used with caution in patients with significant bronchospasm, peripheral vascular disease, or diabetes with severe hypoglycemic episodes.

F. **Calcium Antagonists.** Calcium antagonists block or alter cell membrane calcium flux and are useful agents in diabetic patients who require additional drug therapy to lower blood pressure after an ARB (or ACE inhibitor) and a diuretic. In the SYST-EUR trial, long-acting dihydropyridines reduced fatal and nonfatal cardiac events, including sudden death, by 26% and stroke by 42% at 2 years in older patients with isolated systolic hypertension (Lancet 1997;350:757–64); benefits were especially pronounced in diabetic subjects, with reductions in overall mortality of 55%, cardiovascular mortality of 76%, and stroke of 73% (Lancet 1998;351:1755–62). Four recent hypertension megatrials using amlodipine have confirmed the efficacy and safety of calcium antagonists for hypertension. In the Antihypertensive and Lipid Lowering treatment to prevent Heart Attack Trial (ALLHAT), there was no difference in combined fatal coronary heart disease and nonfatal MI (or in the risk of cancer or GI bleeding) at 4.8 years among 33,357 hypertensive patients (36% with diabetes) randomized to amlodipine, lisinopril, or chlorthalidone (JAMA 2002;288:2981–97). In the Valsartan Antihypertensive Long-term Use Evaluation (VALUE), there was no difference in fatal and nonfatal cardiac events at 4.2 years among 15,245 high-risk hypertensive patients (32% with diabetes) randomized to amlodipine or valsartan, and the amlodipine-based regimen was associated with greater reductions in blood pressure at 1 month, 6 months, and 1 year (Lancet 2004;363:2022–31). In the Anglo-Scandinavian Cardiac Outcomes Trial-Blood Pressure Lowering Arm (ASCOT-BPLA), the amlodipine-based regimen (perindopril added as needed) resulted in better blood pressure control, fewer major cardiovascular events, and less new-onset diabetes than the atenolol-based regimen (bendroflumethiazide added as needed) at 5.5 years among 19,257 high-risk hypertensive patients (23% with diabetes) (Lancet 2005;366:895-906). In the Conduit Artery Function Evaluation (CAFE), a substudy of ASCOT, the amlodipine-based regimen resulted in lower (4.3 mmHg) central aortic systolic blood pressure and lower (3.0 mmHg) central aortic pulse pressure than the atenolol-based regimen despite nearly identical brachial blood pressure between the two study groups (Circulation 2006;113:1213-25). The Avoiding Cardiovascular Events in Combination Therapy in Patients Living with Hypertension (ACCOMPLISH) trial was the first major outcomes trial to evaluate single-tablet combination therapy for hypertension. A total of 11,462 high-risk hypertensive patients (with heart disease, renal disease, or other target organ damage) were randomized to either amlodipine plus benazepril (5/40) or to benazepril plus hydrochlorothiazide (HCTZ) (40/12.5). Sixty percent of patients had diabetes. At a mean follow-up of 39 months, therapy with amlodipine/benazepril reduced cardiovascular morbidity and mortality by 20%, compared to therapy with benazepril/HCTZ, despite similar reductions in blood pressure (presented at the American College of Cardiology meeting, March, 2008, Chicago, IL) Once-daily, fixed-dose combination pills (e.g., calcium antagonist in combination with an ARB, ACE inhibitor, or diuretic) may improve patient compliance by reducing pill burden. A combination pill consisting of amlodipine and atorvastatin (Caduet) is available for the treatment of hypertension and dyslipidemia. Nondihydropyridines should be avoided in patients with severe LV dysfunction, mild to moderate LV dysfunction receiving beta-blockers, sick sinus syndrome, or high-degree AV block. Because of concerns about edema, dihydropyridines should be avoided or used at low initial doses in patients receiving thiazolidinediones.

G. Vasodilators. These drugs enter vascular smooth muscle cells to cause direct vasodilation, in contrast to antihypertensive agents that vasodilate by inhibiting hormonal vasoconstrictor mechanisms (e.g., ACE inhibitors), preventing calcium entry into cells that initiate constriction (e.g., calcium antagonists), or blocking alpha-receptor–mediated vasoconstriction (e.g., alpha-1 blockers). Oral direct vasodilators include hydralazine and minoxidil; intravenous agents include hydralazine, nitroprusside, nitroglycerin, and diazoxide. Hydralazine is used infrequently as an antihypertensive agent, although it may be used in conjunction with isosorbide dinitrate as an alternative to angiotensin II receptor blockers in patients with systolic heart failure who are intolerant of ACE inhibitors. The combination of isosorbide and hydralazine in African-American patients has been shown to be efficacious. Hydralazine has also been used to treat the hypertension of eclampsia. Adverse effects include tachycardia, angina, headache, dizziness, fluid retention, nasal congestion, lupus-like syndrome, and hepatitis. Minoxidil has become a mainstay for severe hypertension associated with renal insufficiency. Adverse effects include tachycardia, angina, fluid retention, pericardial effusion, and hirsutism. To be fully effective, these direct vasodilators should generally be administered in combination with diuretics and beta blockers. Nitroprusside and nitroglycerin are used for hypertensive crisis.

Chapter 9

Other Measures to Reduce Atherothrombosis

Antiplatelet Therapy

A. Overview. Atherothrombotic vascular disease is a dynamic, progressive process of arterial injury, thrombosis, and repair. The resulting atherosclerotic plaque progresses through phases leading to progressive stenosis or acute plaque rupture and intravascular thrombosis, the common underlying mechanism of ischemic stroke, unstable angina, and acute MI (Figure 9.1). Platelet adhesion, activation, and aggregation are central to arterial thrombosis, and antiplatelet therapy has been shown to reduce ischemic stroke, nonfatal MI, and vascular death by 25% in high-risk patients (BMJ 2002;324:71-86). Type 2 diabetic subjects have hyperactive platelets that aggregate more readily in response to platelet agonists, greatly increasing the risk of arterial thrombosis and vascular events.

B. Aspirin. Aspirin exerts its antiplatelet effects by blocking the formation of thromboxane A_2 through irreversible acetylation of platelet cyclooxygenase (Figure 9.2). Enzyme inhibition lasts for the lifespan of the platelet ($\sim$ 10 days). Aspirin does not prevent atherosclerosis, platelet adhesion, or platelet aggregation in response to ADP, collagen, thrombin, or epinephrine. The Antithrombotic Trialists' Collaborative (ATC) overview of randomized trials of antiplatelet therapy, comprising more than 210,000 patients in 287 studies, found that aspirin reduced the risk of vascular events in high-risk patients by 22% (BMJ 2002;324:71-86). It was estimated that when aspirin is used for secondary prevention, 38 $\pm$ 12 vascular events would be prevented per 1000 diabetic patients. In the Early Treatment Diabetic Retinopathy Study (ETDRS), aspirin (650 mg/d) reduced the risk of MI at 5 years by 26% (9.1% vs. 12.3% for placebo, p = 0.04) (JAMA 1992;268:1292-1300). There was no increase

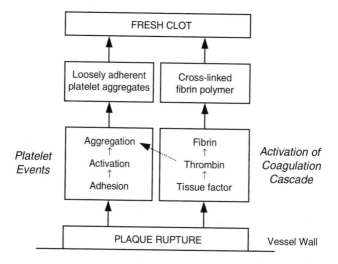

Figure 9.1. Pathophysiology of Atherothrombotic Vascular Disease

Intravascular thrombosis is central to the pathogenesis of acute coronary syndromes and acute ischemic stroke. Plaque rupture exposes circulating blood to vessel wall contents, which rapidly induces clot formation via activation of two complementary systems: platelets and the coagulation cascade. The mechanism of action of antiplatelet agents is shown in Figure 9.2.

in vitreous or retinal hemorrhage in diabetic patients with established retinopathy receiving aspirin in this study. In the Hypertension Optimal Treatment (HOT) study, aspirin (75 mg/d) reduced the risk of major cardiovascular events (MI, stroke, or cardiovascular death) by 15% and MI by 36% in hypertensive diabetic patients (Lancet 1998;351:1755-62).

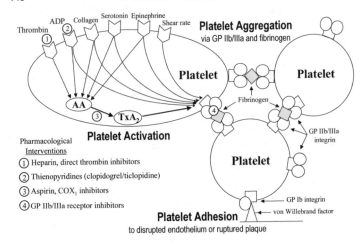

Figure 9.2. Mechanism of Antiplatelet Therapy

AA = arachidonic acid, ADP = adenosine diphosphate, COX = cyclooxygenase, GP = glycoprotein, TXA$_2$ = thromboxane A$_2$. Plaque rupture induces platelets to proceed through adhesion, activation, and aggregation. Platelet adhesion is initiated by the binding of von Willebrand factor (vWF), an adhesive glycoprotein released from the injured vessel wall, to the platelet glycoprotein (GP) Ib receptor. Platelets are exposed to multiple agonists at the same time (ADP, TXA$_2$, epinephrine, thrombin, serotonin, collagen), which trigger a series of events within the platelet, including increased cytosolic calcium, cell shape changes, phosphorylation of proteins, release of granules and lysosomes, arachidonic acid metabolism, and conformational change in the GP IIb/IIIa receptor complex so that it becomes expressed and active on the platelet surface. 50,000-80,000 GP IIb/IIIa receptors reside on the surface of activated platelets. Fibrinogen is the most important ligand of the GP IIb/IIIa receptor and can bind two GP IIa/IIIb receptors simultaneously, creating a molecular platelet-to-platelet bridge. Aspirin blocks the formation of thromboxane A$_2$ through irreversible acetylation of platelet cyclooxygenase. Clopidogrel and ticlopidine irreversibly modify the platelet ADP receptor, interfering with binding of ADP to its receptor and ADP-mediated activation of the GP IIb/IIIa receptor. Dipyridamole is a phosphodiesterase inhibitor that raises platelet levels of cyclic AMP. Adapted from: Peterson M, Dangas G, Fuster V, in: *The Manual of Interventional Cardiology, 3rd ed.,* Physicians' Press, Royal Oak, MI.

Among diabetic physicians in the US Physicians Health Study, a primary prevention trial, low-dose aspirin (325 mg every other day) reduced the risk of MI by 61% (4% vs. 10.1% for placebo). These data establish the important role of aspirin for primary and secondary prevention of cardiovascular events in diabetic patients. Recommendations from the American Diabetes Association regarding the use of aspirin are shown in Table 9.1. The optimal dose of aspirin is not known, although ATC found that doses of 75-150 mg/d seem to be as effective as higher doses for long-term therapy. Doses in excess of 325 mg/d are associated with increased risk of gastrointestinal bleeding in a dose-dependent fashion. Low-dose aspirin (75-81 mg/d) should be considered for patients with a history of serious bleeding, especially from the gastrointestinal tract. Many patients with coronary artery disease, prior stroke, or type 2 diabetes are aspirin-resistant (Circulation 2000;18:II-418; Thromb Haemost 2002;88:711-5), which may increase the risk of recurrent vascular events (Circulation 2002;105:1650-5; Thromb Res 1993;71:397-403). Although methods for detecting these patients are not generally available, they may respond to higher aspirin doses (162-325 mg/d).

C. **Clopidogrel.** Clopidogrel is an inhibitor of ADP-induced platelet activation and subsequent aggregation, acting by irreversible binding to the platelet $P2Y_{12}$ receptor and of the subsequent ADP-mediated activation of the platelet GP IIb/IIIa receptor complex. Clopidogrel irreversibly modifies the platelet ADP receptor so that platelets exposed to clopidogrel are affected for the remainder of their lifespan. Compared to ticlopidine, another thienopyridine derivative, clopidogrel has a longer duration of action, faster onset of action, and is better tolerated due to fewer gastrointestinal symptoms and adverse hematologic effects (Thromb Haemost 1996;76:939-43; Platelets 1993;4:252-61). In the Clopidogrel vs. Aspirin in Patients at Risk for Ischemic Events (CAPRIE) trial, 19,185 patients with atherosclerotic vascular disease (MI

Table 9.1. Aspirin Therapy in Diabetes: Recommendations from the America Diabetes Association

1. Use aspirin therapy (75-162 mg/d) as a secondary prevention strategy in diabetic men and women with evidence of atherosclerotic vascular disease (history of myocardial infarction, vascular bypass procedure, stroke or transient ischemic attack, peripheral vascular disease, claudication, or angina).

2. Use of aspirin therapy (75-162 mg/d) as a primary prevention strategy in type 1 diabetic subjects and in type 2 diabetic subjects at increased cardiovascular risk, including those who are > 40 years of age or who have additional cardiovascular risk factors:
    *   A family history of cardiovascular disease
    *   Cigarette smoking
    *   Hypertension
    *   Albuminuria
    *   Dyslipidemia

3. Combination therapy with aspirin plus other antiplatelet agents (e.g., clopidogrel) should be used in patients with severe and progressive cardiovascular disease

4. People with aspirin allergy, bleeding tendency, anticoagulant therapy, recent gastrointestinal bleeding, and clinically active hepatic disease are not ideal candidates for aspirin therapy. The risks and benefits of aspirin must be carefully considered in these individuals; if aspirin is utilized, the dose should be kept low (81 mg daily).

5. Aspirin therapy is not recommended for patients under the age of 21 years because of the increased risk of Reye's syndrome associated with aspirin use in this population.

Adapted from: Standards of Medical Care in Diabetes, the American Diabetes Association. Diabetes Care 2008;31(suppl 1):S12-S55.

within 35 days, ischemic stroke within 6 months, or established peripheral arterial disease) were randomized to clopidogrel (75 mg/d) or aspirin (325 mg/d). At a mean follow-up of 1.9 years, clopidogrel was more effective than aspirin at reducing the combined endpoint of stroke, MI, or vascular death (relative risk reduction 8.7%; p = 0.043) (Lancet

1996;348:1329). Among 3866 patients with type 2 diabetes in CAPRIE, the absolute risk reduction for the primary endpoint was 2.1%, which was larger than the 0.9% reduction seen in a group without diabetes (Am J Cardiol 2002;90:625-8). Clopidogrel resulted in slightly fewer bleeding complications, and there was no difference in the incidence of severe neutropenia between groups. Clopidogrel is approved for the reduction of atherothrombotic events (MI, ischemic stroke, vascular death) in patients with recent MI, recent stroke, or established peripheral arterial disease, and is an excellent choice for high-risk diabetics who require antiplatelet therapy, particularly those intolerant of or allergic to aspirin or who have a cardiovascular event while taking aspirin. The safety profile of clopidogrel is similar to aspirin and better than ticlopidine, with a rare incidence (~ 4 per million) of thrombotic thrombocytopenic purpura (N Engl J Med 2000;342:1773-7).

D. **Combination Aspirin Plus Clopidogrel.** Ex-vivo platelet aggregation studies and recent clinical trials have shown that utilizing two antiplatelet agents with different mechanisms of action is more effective at preventing platelet aggregation and vascular events than single-agent therapy. This was also shown in several clinical trials, including the Clopidogrel in Unstable angina to prevent Recurrent Events (CURE) trial (N Engl J Med 2001;345:494-502); the Clopidogrel as Adjunctive Reperfusion Therapy (CLARITY)-TIMI 28 study (ST-elevation MI < 12 hours treated with fibrinolytic therapy [N Engl J Med 2005;352:1179-89]); the Clopidogrel and Metoprolol in Myocardial Infarction Trial (COMMIT) (acute MI < 24 hours not undergoing primary PCI [Lancet 2005;366:1622-1632]); and the Clopidogrel for the Reduction of Events During Observation (CREDO) trial (elective PCI [JAMA 2002;288:2411-20]). In contrast, no benefit was observed for combination aspirin plus clopidogrel in the Management of ATherothrombosis with Clopidogrel in High-risk patients (MATCH) trial (recent TIA or ischemic stroke at high risk for recurrent ischemic events [Lancet 2004;364:331-337]) or the Clopidogrel for High Atherothrombotic Risk and Ischemic Stabilization Management and Avoidance (CHARISMA) trial (stable vascular disease or multiple risk factors [New Engl J Med 2006;354:1706-17]). Clopidogrel is indicated for use in aspirin-intolerant patients and in patients with severe and progressive cardiovascular disease. Clopidogrel 75 mg/d is also indicated in combination with aspirin for up to 12 months in patients after acute coronary syndrome or percutaneous coronary intervention with stent placement (J Am Coll Cardiol 2006;47:2130-9). Some analyses have suggested that coadministration of atorvastatin inhibits the antiplatelet effects of clopidogrel, but a prospective study designed to examine this potential interaction did not find a significant difference in platelet measures (Ann Intern Med 2004;164:2051-7).

E. **Glycoprotein IIb/IIIa Inhibitors.** GP IIb/IIIa receptor antagonists are the most potent platelet inhibitors available. They exert their antiplatelet effects by blocking the binding of fibrinogen to the GP IIb/IIIa receptor on the platelet surface, the final common pathway of platelet aggregation. GP IIb/IIIa inhibitors block platelet aggregation in response to all platelet agonists (e.g., collagen, thrombin, ADP, epinephrine, thromboxane A_2). Abciximab is a monoclonal antibody and noncompetitive inhibitor that binds 1:1 to the GP IIb/IIIa receptor molecule to induce a conformational change that renders the fibrinogen-binding site of the receptor inactive. Eptifibatide and tirofiban are small-molecule competitive inhibitors of the RGD tripeptide-binding domain of the GP IIb/IIIa receptor. In a pooled analysis of 6458 diabetic subjects enrolled into one of six randomized trials of GP IIb/IIIa inhibitors vs. placebo for medical management of non-ST-elevation acute coronary syndromes (PURSUIT, PRISM, PRISM-PLUS, GUSTO-V, PARAGON A, PARAGON B), GP IIb/IIIa inhibitors reduced 30-day mortality by 26% (4.6% vs. 6.2%, p = 0.007). In a pooled analysis of 1462 diabetic subjects enrolled into one of three randomized trials of GP IIb/IIIa inhibitors vs. placebo as adjuncts to percutaneous coronary intervention (EPIC, EPILOG, EPISTENT), abciximab reduced 1-year mortality by 44% (2.5% vs. 4.5%, p = 0.031) (S. Marso, personal communication). Ongoing trials will help determine the optimal GP IIb/IIIa inhibitor for non-ST-elevation ACS and elective PCI and the role for adjunctive antithrombin therapy (unfractionated heparin, low-molecular-weight heparin, direct thrombin inhibitors) and other antiplatelet agents (aspirin, clopidogrel).

ACE Inhibitors / ARBs

Angiotensin converting enzyme (ACE) inhibitors block the conversion of angiotensin I to angiotensin II and inhibit the breakdown of bradykinin, resulting in physiologic benefits that confer unique cardioprotective and renoprotective properties to this class of drugs. ACE inhibitors have been shown to improve prognosis following coronary revascularization procedures and in a wide variety of cardiovascular disorders, including hypertension, heart failure, asymptomatic LV dysfunction, MI, proteinuric nephropathy, and diabetic nephropathy/retinopathy/neuropathy. Angiotensin receptor blockers (ARBs) are effective antihypertensive agents with proven cardioprotective properties in patients with hypertensive LVH, heart failure, and acute MI. They also exert renoprotective effects, reducing proteinuria and slowing the deterioration in renal function in diabetic nephropathy. Compelling data from the HOPE, EUROPA and ON-TARGET trials demonstrate an important role for ACE inhibitors and for ARBs in the prevention of atherothrombotic vascular disease and its complications.

A. **HOPE Study.** The Heart Outcomes Prevention Evaluation (HOPE) study randomized 9297 patients $\geq$ 55 years with either atherosclerotic arterial disease (prior MI, prior stroke, or peripheral arterial disease) or diabetes plus one additional risk factor (hypertension, elevated total cholesterol, depressed HDL cholesterol, smoking, or microalbuminuria) to ramipril (10 mg/d) or placebo. At a mean follow-up of 5 years, ramipril reduced the primary composite endpoint of MI, stroke, or death from cardiovascular disease by 22% (14.0% vs. 17.8%, p < 0.001) (N Engl J Med 2000;342:145-53). In addition, death from cardiovascular causes was reduced by 26% (6.1% vs. 8.1%) and all-cause mortality was reduced by 16% (10.4% vs. 12.2%). Significant risk reduction was also noted for MI (20%), stroke (32%), cardiac arrest (38%), revascularization procedures (15%), and patient-reported new-onset diabetes mellitus (34%). (Ramipril did not reduce new-onset diabetes in DREAM.) The beneficial effects of ramipril were observed in patients with and without diabetes, hypertension, or cardiovascular disease and were independent of the effects of concomitant cardiovascular medications (aspirin, beta-blockers, lipid-lowering agents, other blood pressure drugs). Among 3577 diabetics enrolled in HOPE, ramipril reduced the risk of MI, stroke, or cardiovascular death at 4.5 years by 25% compared to placebo (p = 0.0004). Significant risk reduction was noted for death (6.2% vs. 9.7%, p < 0.001), MI (10.2% vs. 12.9%, p = 0.01), stroke (4.2% vs. 6.1%, p = 0.007), and overt nephropathy (6.5% vs. 8.4%, p = 0.027) (Lancet 2000;35:253-9). Ramipril is approved to reduce the risk of MI, stroke, and death from cardiovascular causes in patients 55 years or older at high risk of developing a major cardiovascular event because of a history of coronary artery disease, stroke, peripheral arterial disease, or diabetes that is accompanied by at least one other cardiovascular risk factor (hypertension, elevated total cholesterol levels, low HDL levels, cigarette smoking, or documented microalbuminuria). The recommended starting dose is 2.5 mg once daily for 1 week, followed by 5 mg once daily for the next 3 weeks, then increased as tolerated to a maintenance dose of 10 mg once a day (which may be given in 2 divided doses for patients with hypertension or recent MI).

B. **EUROPA and PEACE Trials.** The European Trial with Perindopril in Stable Coronary Artery Disease (EUROPA) was undertaken to evaluate the role of ACE inhibitors on cardiovascular risk in low-risk patients ≥ 18 years without clinical heart failure and with stable coronary heart disease (prior MI > 3 months or coronary revascularization > 6 months before screening, ≥ 70% coronary artery stenosis on angiography, or men with a history of chest pain and a positive stress test). 12% of patients had diabetes (vs. 38% in HOPE), 27% had hypertension (vs. 47% in HOPE), 81% had no angina (vs. 20% in HOPE), and 17% had mild angina. 12,218 men and women were randomized to perindopril 8 mg/d (after tolerating 4 mg/d x 2 weeks) or placebo; half the usual dose was given to patients > 70 years of age. At a mean follow-up of 4.2 years, perindopril reduced the primary composite endpoint of cardiovascular death, MI, or cardiac arrest by 20% (8.0% vs. 9.9%, p < 0.0003) (Lancet 2003;362:782-8). The beneficial effects of perindopril were observed in all age groups (≤ 55 years, 56-65 years, > 65 years) and in patients with and without diabetes, hypertension, or prior MI. Benefits were independent of the effects of concomitant cardiovascular medications (aspirin, beta-blockers, lipid-lowering agents, blood pressure drugs). In the Prevention of Events with Angiotensin Converting Enzyme Inhibitors (PEACE) trial, lower-risk patients (compared to HOPE and EUROPA) with stable coronary artery disease and normal/near normal left ventricular function being treated aggressively with coronary revascularization and risk factor modification derived no benefit from the addition of trandolapril at 4.8 years (N Engl J Med 2004;351:2058-68). In this trial, average baseline ejection fraction was 58%, creatinine and cholesterol levels were normal, BP was 133/78 mmHg, and the annualized death rate was only 1.6%, similar to age/sex-matched general population.

C. **ONTARGET Trial.** In the Ongoing Telmisartan Alone and in Combination with Ramipril Global Endpoint Trial (ONTARGET), patients with vascular disease or high-risk diabetes without heart failure were randomized to either telmisartan 80 mg/d (n = 8542), ramipril 10 mg/d (n = 8576), or combination therapy with both drugs (n = 8502). At a median follow-up of 56 months, the primary outcome – cardiovascular death, MI, stroke, or hospitalization for heart failure – was equivalent in all 3 groups (~ 16%). Compared to ramipril, telmisartan was associated with less cough (1.1% vs. 4.2%, p = 0.001) and less angioedema (0.1% vs. 0.3%, p = 0.01). The combination of the two drugs was associated with more adverse events without an increase in clinical benefit (N Engl J Med 2008;358:1547-59).

D. **Recommendations.** ACE inhibitors and ARBs are generally safe, well-tolerated, and affordable. Diabetic patients with hypertension, atherosclerotic vascular disease or age ≥ 55 years with at least one other cardiovascular risk factor (hypertension, elevated total cholesterol, low HDL cholesterol, cigarette smoking, microalbuminuria) should be considered for therapy with either an ACE inhibitor or an ARB. Potential mechanisms for improved cardiovascular prognosis include reductions in left ventricular hypertrophy and arterial wall stress (JAMA 1996;275:1507-13), blood pressure lowering, and improved endothelial function (J Am Coll Cardiol 2000;35:60-6).

Fish Oil

In the GISSI Prevention Study of 11,324 patients with prior MI, 1 gm/d (850 mg of DHA and EPA) of fish oil, a dose too low to affect lipid levels, reduced total mortality by 20% at 3.5 years, including a 45% reduction in sudden cardiac death (Lancet 1999;354:447-55). Similar benefits were seen in DART, in which men with prior MI who were instructed to eat fatty fish at least twice weekly or take a fish oil supplement had a 29% reduction in total mortality (Lancet 1989;2:757-61). In the JELIS trial, 18,600 adults with hypercholesterolemia were randomized to statin alone or statin plus EPA 2 gm/d. The statin plus EPA group experienced a 19% reduction (p = 0.01) in major adverse coronary events at 5 years (Lancet 2007;369:1090-98). Consumption of fish and omega-3 fatty acids has also been shown to reduce the risk of CHD in otherwise healthy persons and is an important component of the Mediterranean-style diet (Chapter 4). Individuals with diabetes should be instructed to eat at least 2 servings of fish high in omega-3 fats per week. High-dose fish oil supplements (3-10 gm/d) can be used to lower triglyceride levels (Chapter 7). Lovaza (formerly Omacor), which contains highly purified omega-3 or acid ethyl esters, mainly EPA and DHA (850 mg per 1 gram capsule), has been approved by the FDA for the treatment of triglyceride levels $\geq$ 500 mg/dL at a daily dose of 4 gm/day.

Alcohol

Most observational studies show that people who consume 2-14 drinks per week (ideally 1 drink per day) have lower rates of cardiovascular events and all-cause mortality compared to nondrinkers. The benefits of moderate alcohol intake are even more impressive in diabetic individuals compared to the general population because of the higher incidence of cardiac events in diabetes and the ability of alcohol to lower insulin resistance, raise HDL-C, and decrease platelet aggregation. One drink per day has also been shown to lower the risk of developing type 2 diabetes; it will also lower postprandial glucose levels by 20-30% in individuals with or without diabetes. One drink is defined as 12 ounces of beer, 5.5 ounces of wine, or 1.5 ounces of 80-

proof distilled liquor (spirits). However, blood pressure and triglycerides rise proportionately with alcohol intake of more than 3 drinks per day; at intake above this level of alcohol consumption, the reduction in cardiovascular mortality is offset by the increased risk of cancer, strokes, and accidents. Optimal intake of alcohol is not more than 2 drinks daily for men or 1 drink daily for women. Although light to moderate alcohol consumption (up to 1 oz ethanol per day) has been associated with a lower risk of CHD, it is not recommended as a therapeutic agent because of possible deleterious effects, such as hypertriglyceridemia, hypertension and increased risk of breast and other cancers, and because it is difficult to predict who might be at risk for alcohol abuse.

Influenza and Pneumococcal Vaccination

Influenza epidemics occur most often during the winter months and are responsible for more than 40,000 deaths each year in the U.S. alone. To prevent hospitalization and death, the Advisory Committee on Immunization Practices (ACIP) recommends annual influenza vaccination for higher-risk individuals, including those with type 2 diabetes (www.cdc.gov). Patients with type 2 diabetes should also receive pneumococcal vaccine (Pneumovax) to reduce the risk for pneumococcal pneumonia (primary dose: 0.5 mL). A one-time booster dose is recommended for individuals ≥ 65 years of age if the primary dose was received before age 65 and it has been > 5 years since the primary dose was given. A booster dose is also recommended for diabetic subjects with the nephrotic syndrome, chronic kidney disease, or other immunocompromised conditions (e.g., post-transplantation).

Chapter 10. Clinical Trials

Table 10.1. Diabetes Care Trials

Trial	Design	Results
ACCORD: Action to Control Cardiovascular Risk in Diabetes (N Engl J Med 2008;358:2545-2559)	10,251 type 2 diabetic patients (mean age 62.2 years, mean HbA_{1c} 8.1%) with established cardiovascular disease or additional cardiovascular risk factors were randomized to intensive (HbA_{1c} < 6.0%) vs. standard glycemic control (HbA_{1c} of 7.0-7.9%).	After 3.5 years, the trial was suspended due to significantly more deaths from any cause in the intensive therapy group compared to the standard therapy group ($p = 0.04$). Additionally, the use of intensive therapy did not significantly reduce the primary outcome of major cardiovascular events (cardiovascular death, nonfatal MI, or nonfatal stroke) ($p = 0.16$). Both treatment groups had far fewer adverse cardiovascular events than expected. Hypoglycemia requiring assistance and weight gain > 10 kg occurred more often in the intensive therapy group ($p < 0.001$).
ADOPT: A Diabetes Outcome Progression Trial (N Engl J Med 2006;355:2427-43)	4,360 treatment-naive patients with type 2 diabetes were randomized to 4 years of monotherapy with rosiglitazone, metformin, or glyburide. Primary outcome: time to monotherapy failure (FPG > 180 mg/dL).	Cumulative incidence of monotherapy failure at 5 years was significantly less for rosiglitazone (15%) than for either metformin (21%) or glyburide (34%), representing risk reductions of 32% and 63%, respectively ($p < 0.001$ for both comparisons).

See p. 1 for abbreviations

Table 10.1. Diabetes Care Trials

Trial	Design	Results
ADVANCE: Action in Diabetes and Vascular Disease: Preterax and Diamicron Modified Release Controlled Evaluation (N Engl J Med 2008;358:2560-2572)	11,140 patients age ≥ 55 years with type 2 diabetes diagnosed after age 30 and with cardiovascular disease or at least one cardiovascular risk factor were randomized to intensive (HbA$_{1c}$ of 6.5% or less) vs. standard glucose control (HbA$_{1c}$ ~ 7.0%). Primary endpoints were a composite of major macrovascular events (cardiovascular death, nonfatal MI, or nonfatal stroke) and major microvascular events (new or worsening nephropathy or retinopathy).	At 5 years, the mean HbA$_{1c}$ was 6.5% in the intensive glycemic group vs. 7.3% in the standard group ($p < 0.001$). This reduction was associated with a 10% relative risk reduction for major macrovascular and microvascular complications (18.1% vs. 20.0%, $p = 0.01$) and a 14% relative risk reduction for major microvascular events (9.4% vs. 10.9%, $p = 0.01$), primarily due to a 21% reduction in nephropathy (4.1% vs. 5.2%, $p = 0.006$). There was no significant difference between groups for major macrovascular events such as MI or stroke ($p = 0.32$). A 9% decrease in new microalbuminuria ($p = 0.02$) was also documented in the intensive glycemic group.
DCCT: Diabetes Control and Complications Trial (N Engl J Med 2005;353:2643-2653)	1,441 patients aged 13-39 years with type 1 diabetes were randomized to intensive blood glucose control vs. normal care. Follow-up: 20 years.	Intensive glucose control reduced the combined endpoint of major macrovascular events by 50% ($p = NS$). MI was 5 times more frequent with conventional treatment (0.29 vs. 0.06 events/100 patients years, $p = 0.065$).

Table 10.1. Diabetes Care Trials

Trial	Design	Results
DIGAMI: Diabetes Mellitus Insulin Glucose Infusion in Acute Myocardial Infarction (J Am Coll Cardiol 1995;26:57-65)	620 patients with diabetes and acute MI were randomized to insulin and glucose infusion (followed by SQ insulin post-discharge for 3 months) vs. conventional therapy.	Insulin treatment was associated with a 29% decrease in mortality at 1 year (p = 0.027).
DPP: Diabetes Prevention Project (N Engl J Med 2002;346:393-403)	3,234 patients with elevated fasting and post-load glucose levels (but not diabetes) were randomized to lifestyle intervention (≥ 150 minutes of exercise/week and a weight-loss diet), metformin (850 mg bid), or placebo.	Lifestyle modification decreased the incidence of new diabetes by 58% (p < 0.001 vs. placebo), and metformin decreased the incidence of new diabetes by 31% (p < 0.001 vs. placebo) over 2.8 years of follow-up.
DREAM: Diabetes Reduction Assessment with Ramipril and Rosiglitazone Medication (Lancet 2006;368:1096-1105)	5,269 patients aged ≥ 30 years with IFG (mean FPG 104 mg/dL) or IGT (mean 2-hour post-challenge blood glucose 156 mg/dL) were randomized to rosiglitazone 8 mg/d or placebo in a factorial design. Primary endpoint: new diabetes or death. Follow-up: 3 years.	Rosiglitazone reduced the primary endpoint by 60% (11.6% vs. 26.0%, p < 0.0001). Additionally, reversion to normoglycemia occurred more often with rosiglitazone (50.5% vs. 30.3% for placebo, p < 0.0001). Cardiovascular event rates were similar, except for CHF (0.5% for rosiglitazone vs. 0.1% for placebo, p = 0.01).
Finnish Diabetes Prevention Study (N Engl J Med 2001;344:1343-1350)	522 overweight men and women (mean age 55 years) were randomized to a control group or intensive counseling for weight control, saturated fat intake, fiber intake, and physical activity. Mean follow-up: 3.2 years.	Intensive counseling and lifestyle modification led to a 58% decrease in the risk of developing new diabetes (11% vs. 23%, p < 0.001). Amount of weight loss was greater in the intervention group (3.5 kg vs. 0.8 kg, p < 0.001).

See p. 1 for abbreviations

Table 10.1. Diabetes Care Trials

Trial	Design	Results
Gomez-Perez et al. Efficacy and Safety of Rosiglitazone plus Metformin in Mexicans with Type 2 Diabetes (Diabetes Metab Res Rev 2002;18:127-134)	116 Mexican patients with diabetes and poor glucose control on metformin alone were randomized to rosiglitazone 2 or 4 mg bid or placebo in addition to metformin 2.5 g/d. Follow-up: 24 weeks.	HbA_{1c} decreased with rosiglitazone therapy in addition to metformin (2 mg bid: –0.7%, p = 0.005; 4 mg bid: –1.2%, p < 0.001). It was unchanged in the placebo group. Mean fasting glucose also decreased with rosiglitazone (p < 0.002). Total-to-HDL ratio remained unchanged.
Indian Diabetes Prevention Program (Diabetologia 2006;49:289-97)	421 men and 110 women with IGT were randomized to a control group, a lifestyle modification group, a metformin group, or a metformin plus lifestyle modification group x 30 months.	Compared to control, the risk of new-onset diabetes was reduced by lifestyle modification (28.5% reduction, p = 0.018), metformin (26.4% reduction, p = 0.029), and lifestyle modification plus metformin (28.2% reduction, p = 0.022).
MRFIT: Multiple Risk Factor Intervention Trial (Diabetes Care 1993;16:435-444)	347,978 men (5,163 taking medication for diabetes) were enrolled and followed for a mean of 12 years to compare the risk of CV death in men with and without diabetes and to assess predictors of CV mortality.	There were 160 deaths per 10,000 person-years in the diabetes group compared with 53.2 in the non-diabetic group. After adjusting for age, race, cholesterol, BP and smoking, mortality remained three times greater in men with diabetes.

See p. 1 for abbreviations

Table 10.1. Diabetes Care Trials

Trial	Design	Results
Steno-2 Study (N Engl J Med 2003;348:383-393)	160 diabetic patients with microalbuminuria (mean age 55.1 years) were randomized to conventional treatment to Danish Diabetes Association guidelines or to intensive treatment (behavior modification; medical therapy for hyperglycemia, hypertension, dyslipidemia, and microalbuminuria; and aspirin). Follow-up: 7.8 years.	Intensive therapy led to significant reductions in CV disease (53%), nephropathy (61%), retinopathy (58%), and autonomic neuropathy (63%). There were significant reductions in HbA_{1c}, BP, total cholesterol, triglycerides, and urinary albumin excretion rate.
STOP-NIDDM: Study to Prevent NIDDM (Lancet 2002;359:2072-2077)	1,429 patients with impaired glucose tolerance were randomized to acarbose 100 mg tid or placebo. Follow-up: 3.9 years.	Acarbose reduced the risk of new diabetes by 25% (p = 0.0015), new hypertension by 24% (p = 0.0059), and CV events by 40% (p = 0.027).
TRIPOD: Troglitazone in the Prevention of Diabetes (Diabetes 2002;51:2796-2803)	266 Hispanic women with a history of gestational diabetes were randomized to troglitazone 400 mg/d or placebo. Follow-up: 2.5 years.	Troglitazone reduced the incidence of new diabetes by 56% (p < 0.01) and maintained lower incidence off drug for 10 months
UKPDS 33: United Kingdom Prospective Diabetes Study (Lancet 1998;352:837-853)	3,867 men and women with newly diagnosed diabetes were randomized to intensive blood glucose control (insulin or a sulfonylurea) or conventional care (diet modification). Follow-up: 10 years.	HbA_{1c} was 11% lower in the intensive care group (7.0% vs. 7.9%). This was associated with a 12% lower risk for any diabetes-related endpoint (p = 0.029) and non-significant reductions in diabetes-related death (10%, p = 0.34) and all-cause mortality (6%, p = 0.44).

See p. 1 for abbreviations

Table 10.1. Diabetes Care Trials

Trial	Design	Results
UKPDS 34: United Kingdom Prospective Diabetes Study (Lancet 1998;352: 854-865)	753 men and women with newly diagnosed diabetes and obesity (> 120% ideal body weight) were randomized to intensive blood glucose control with metformin or conventional care (diet modification). Follow-up: 10.7 years.	Metformin reduced the risk of diabetes-related complications by 32% (p = 0.002), diabetes-related death by 42% (p = 0.017), and all-cause mortality by 36% (p = 0.11). Secondary analysis showed metformin was more effective in reducing endpoints than sulfonylureas or insulin.
UKPDS 35: United Kingdom Prospective Diabetes Study (BMJ 2000;321: 405-412)	4,585 men and women with diabetes were randomized to intensive blood glucose control (insulin or a sulfonylurea) or conventional care (diet modification). Follow-up: 10 years.	Each 1% decrease in HbA_{1c} reduced the risk of diabetes-related complications by 21% (p < 0.0001), diabetes-related death by 21% (p < 0.0001), MI by 14% (p < 0.0001), and microvascular complications by 37% (p < 0.0001). No threshold of risk was observed for any endpoint.
VADT: Veterans Affairs Diabetes Trial (Presented at the American Diabetes Association Scientific Sessions, San Francisco, CA, June, 2008)	1791 patients with type 2 diabetes were randomized to intensive or standard glycemic control. At enrollment, more than 40% of participants had suffered prior cardiovascular events, and most were obese with abnormal lipid profiles and hypertension. Mean HbA_{1c} was 9.5% at baseline, and was reduced to 6.9% and 8.4% in the intensive and standard therapy groups, respectively.	At 7.5 years, there was no reduction in the primary endpoint – stroke, MI, CHF, and CV death – in the intensive glycemic group. However, it was noted that lowering blood glucose to near normal levels may reduce the risk of major adverse CV events if therapy is initiated relatively soon after diagnosis, esp. in those with less advanced atherosclerosis, and if episodes of severe hypoglycemia can be avoided. Both treatment groups had far fewer CV events than expected.

See p. 1 for abbreviations

Table 10.1. Diabetes Care Trials

Trial	Design	Results
XENDOS: Xenical in the Prevention of Diabetes in Obese Subjects (Rev Med Liege 2002;57:617-621)	3,304 obese patients (BMI ≥ 30 kg/m² were randomized to orlistat or lifestyle modification for weight loss and to evaluate its effect on the incidence of diabetes. Follow-up: 4 years.	Orlistat treatment led to a 37% relative reduction in new diabetes (6.2% vs. 9.0%, p = 0.003). The group with impaired glucose tolerance and weight loss had a greater absolute reduction (19% vs. 29%, p < 0.005).

Table 10.2. Diabetes Epidemiology Studies

Trial	Design	Results
ARIC: Atherosclerosis Risk in Communities Study (Ann Intern Med 2000;81-91)	1,676 patients aged 45-64 with diabetes and no known CHD were followed for 8 years to examine the association of traditional and nontraditional CHD risk factors in patients with diabetes.	186 (11.1%) developed CHD, and risk was related to traditional risk factors (high LDL, low HDL, hypertension, smoking). Markers of inflammation (low albumin, high fibrinogen, high von Willebrand factor, high leukocyte count) also correlated with development of CHD.
DECODE: Diabetes Epidemiology Collaborative Analysis of Diagnostic Criteria in Europe (Lancet 1999;354:617-621)	Over 25,000 patients from 13 European trials were analyzed to compare the mortality of patients meeting ADA criteria for diabetes (fasting plasma glucose > 126 mg/dL only) with those meeting the WHO criteria (2-hour post-load glucose > 200 mg/dL).	Using ADA criteria, the hazard ratio for death was 1.81 for men and 1.79 for women (vs. normal glucose tolerance). For those meeting WHO criteria, the hazard ratio for death was 2.02 in men and 2.77 in women. Those with normal fasting glucose and impaired 2-hour glucose tolerance had the greatest risk of death.

See p. 1 for abbreviations

Table 10.2. Diabetes Epidemiology Studies

Trial	Design	Results
Norhammer et al. Glucose Metabolism in Patients with Acute MI and no Previous Diagnosis of Diabetes Mellitus (Lancet 2002;359: 2140- 2144)	181 consecutive patients (mean age 63.5 years) who were admitted with acute MI, no known DM, and glucose < 200 mg/dL were given a standard oral glucose tolerance test at discharge and 3 months to define the prevalence of impaired glucose tolerance (IGT).	At hospital discharge, 35% of patients had IGT, and 31% had unrecognized diabetes. At 3 months, 40% had IGT and 25% were diagnosed with diabetes.
Nurses' Health Study (N Engl J Med 2001;345:790-797, Am J Public Health 2000;90:1490- 1415)	84,941 women aged 38-63 years with no history of diabetes or CHD were followed for 10 years to identify factors predisposing to the development of diabetes.	91% of diabetes (n = 3,300) could be attributed to habits and forms of behavior that did not conform to the low-risk pattern (diet rich in whole grains and low in trans-fats and glycemic load, exercise, abstinence from smoking, and ≥ ½ alcoholic beverage daily). Women in the low-risk group had a relative risk of diabetes of 0.09 (95% CI, 0.05 to 0.17).
Physician's Health Study (JAMA 1992;268:63-67)	21,271 male US physicians aged 40-84 years were enrolled and followed for 5 years to assess the effect of vigorous exercise on the development of diabetes.	Those who exercised at least once weekly had a 37% lower incidence of new diabetes than those who exercised less often (p < 0.001).
Physician's Health Study – Diabetic Subgroup (Arch Intern Med 2001;161:242-247)	2,317 male US physicians with diabetes and 815 with both diabetes and CHD aged 40-84 years were enrolled and followed for 5 years to assess the impact of diabetes on all-cause and CHD mortality.	The relative risk for all-cause mortality was 2.3 for men with diabetes and 4.7 for men with diabetes and CHD. The relative risk for CHD death was 3.3 with diabetes, and 12.0 for those with both diabetes and CHD.

See p. 1 for abbreviations

Table 10.2. Diabetes Epidemiology Studies

Trial	Design	Results
Sinha et al. Prevalence of Impaired Glucose Tolerance among Children and Adolescents with Marked Obesity (N Engl J Med 2002:346:820-810)	55 children (aged 4-10 years) and 112 adolescents (aged 11-18 years) with a body mass index greater than the 95th percentile for age and sex underwent 2-hour oral glucose tolerance testing.	Impaired glucose tolerance (fasting plasma glucose < 126 mg/dL and 2-hour plasma glucose 140-200 mg/dL) was detected in 25% of obese children and 22% of obese adolescents.

See p. 1 for abbreviations

Chapter 11

Diabetes Drug Summaries

This section contains prescribing information pertinent to the clinical use of common diabetic medications, as compiled from a variety of sources (see below). The information provided is not exhaustive, and the reader is referred to other drug information references and the manufacturer's product literature for further information. Clinical use of the information provided and any consequences that may arise from its use are the responsibilities of the prescribing physician. The authors, editors, and publisher do not warrant or guarantee the information contained in this section, and do not assume and expressly disclaim any liability for errors or omissions or any consequences that may occur from such. The use of any drug should be preceded by careful review of the package insert, which provides indications and dosing approved by the U.S. Food and Drug Administration. (Package inserts can be found on the websites provided at the end of each drug summary.) Drugs are listed alphabetically by generic name; trade names follow in parentheses. To search by trade name, consult the index. Safety in pregnancy listing is designated by the U.S. Food and Drug Administration's (USFDA) use-in-pregnancy letter code (Table 11.1, next page).

Drug References:
1. American Association of Clinical Endocrinologists and American College of Clinical Endocrinologists. Medical Guidelines for the Management of Diabetes Mellitus: The AACE System of Intensive Diabetes Self-Management – 2002 Update. Endocr Pract 2002;8(Suppl 1).
2. Physician's Desk Reference (PDR), 2008.
3. Drug Facts and Comparisons, 2008.
4. Zangeneh F, Kudva YC, Basu A. Insulin sensitizers. Mayo Clin Proc 2003;78:471-479.
5. DeWitt, DE, Hirsch IB. Outpatient insulin therapy in type 1 diabetes mellitus. JAMA 2003;289:2254-2264.
6. Inzucchi SE. Oral antihyperglycemic therapy for type 2 diabetes. JAMA 2002;287:360-372.
7. Nathan DM. Initial management of glycemia in type 2 diabetes mellitus. N Engl J Med 2002;347:1342-1349.

Table 11.1. USFDA Use-in-Pregnancy Letter Code

Category	Interpretation
A	**Controlled studies show no risk.** Adequate, well-controlled studies in pregnant women have not shown a risk to the fetus in any trimester of pregnancy.
B	**No evidence of risk in humans.** Adequate, well-controlled studies in pregnant women have not shown increased risk of fetal abnormalities despite adverse findings in animals, or, in the absence of adequate human studies, animal studies show no fetal risk. The chance of fetal harm is remote, but remains a possibility.
C	**Risk cannot be ruled out.** Adequate, well-controlled human studies are lacking, and animal studies have shown a risk to the fetus or are lacking. There is a chance of fetal harm if the drug is administered during pregnancy, but potential benefit from use of the drug may outweigh potential risk.
D	**Positive evidence of risk.** Studies in humans or investigational or post-marketing data have demonstrated fetal risk. Nevertheless, potential benefit from use of the drug may outweigh potential risk. For example, the drug may be acceptable if needed in a life-threatening situation or serious disease for which safer drugs cannot be used or are ineffective.
X	**Contraindicated in pregnancy.** Studies in animals or humans or investigational or post-marketing reports have demonstrated positive evidence of fetal abnormalities or risk which clearly outweigh any possible benefit to the patient.

Chapter 11

Diabetes Drug Summaries

Acarbose (Precose)

Class: Alpha-glucosidase inhibitor
Mechanism of Action: These drugs act locally in the small intestine by inhibiting alpha-glucosidase enzymes; this action slows digestion of ingested carbohydrates, delays glucose absorption, and reduces the increase in postprandial blood glucose.
Clinical Effects: Alpha-glucosidase inhibitors cause a 0.5-1% reduction in HbA1c and have no significant effect on fasting blood glucose levels.
Dosage: 25 mg three times/day with the first bite of each main meal. Maintenance dose ranges are 50-100 mg three times/day. Dose adjustments should be made at 4-8 week intervals. Maximum dosage ≤ 60 kg = 50 mg tid; > 60 kg = 100 mg tid.
Renal Impairment: Not recommended in patients with CrCl < 25 mL/min.
Hepatic Impairment: No dosage adjustment necessary.
Contraindications: Major GI disorders, including inflammatory bowel disease, chronic ulceration, malabsorption, or partial intestinal obstruction. Not recommended for use in patients with CrCl < 25 mL/min.
Adverse Effects: Abdominal bloating, flatulence, diarrhea. Adverse GI effects tend to diminish with continued treatment.

Monitoring: HbA1c, FBG, LFT's (every 3 months).
Drug Interactions: Decreased acarbose effect with intestinal adsorbents (charcoal) and digestive enzyme preparations (amylase, pancreatin).
Safety in Pregnancy: B
Comments: Most useful in patients with postprandial hyperglycemia; not associated with hypoglycemia or weight gain. Must use glucose and not complex sugars to reverse hypoglycemia, if it occurs.
Dosage Forms: 25 mg, 50 mg, 100 mg tablets.
Website: www.pdr.net

Colesevelam (Welchol)

Class: Bile acid sequestrant
Mechanism of Action: (1) Type 2 diabetes mellitus: The mechanism by which colesevelam improves glycemic control is unknown. (2) Primary hyperlipidemia: Cholesterol is a precursor of bile acids, which are secreted via the bile from the liver and gallbladder to emulsify intestinal fats and lipids in foods. Colesevelam binds bile acids in the intestine and decreases their reabsorption, resulting in increased bile acid production in the liver; LDL receptors are upregulated to meet the increased need for cholesterol, facilitating clearance of LDL cholesterol

from the circulation. This agent may increase triglycerides, VLDL, and HDL.

Indications: (1) Type 2 diabetes mellitus: as an adjunct to diet and exercise to improve glycemic control; (2) Primary hyperlipidemia: alone or in combination with a statin as an adjunct to diet and exercise for reduction of elevated LDL cholesterol in patients with primary hypercholesterolemia (Type IIa).

Dosage: *Monotherapy:* Usual starting dose is 3 tablets twice daily with meals or 6 tablets once daily with a meal. The dose can be increased to 7 tablets. *Combination therapy:* Doses of 4 to 6 tablets per day have been shown to be safe and effective when coadministered with a statin or when the two drugs are dosed apart. For maximal therapeutic effect, the recommended dose is 3 tablets taken twice daily with meals or 6 tablets taken once daily with a meal.

Contraindications: Bowel obstruction, hypersensitivity.

Adverse Effects: Constipation, N/V/D, abdominal pain, flatulence, headache, fatigue, myalgia, flu syndrome.

Monitoring: Serum cholesterol and triglycerides; HbA1c.

Drug Interactions: This agent may interfere with absorption of vitamins A, D, E, K, and folic acid. No significant effect on bioavailability of digoxin, metoprolol, quinidine, lovastatin, valproic acid, or warfarin.

Dosage Forms: Tablet (625 mg)

Website: www.welchol.com

Exenatide (Byetta)

Class: Incretin mimetic

Mechanism of Action: Incretins, such as glucagon-like peptide-1, enhance glucose-dependent insulin secretion and exhibit other antihyperglycemic actions following their release into the circulation from the gut. Exenatide is an incretin mimetic agent that enhances glucose-dependent insulin secretion by the pancreatic beta-cell, suppresses inappropriately elevated glucagon secretion, and slows gastric emptying.

Clinical Effects: Exenatide, in combination with metformin, a sulfonylurea, or both, reduces HbA1c by 0.4-1.1%, fasting blood glucose by 10-25 mg/dL, 2-hour post-prandial blood glucose by 60-70 mg/dL, and body weight by 0.9-3.6 kg.

Dosage: Starting dose is 5 mcg twice a day, given within the 60-minute period before the morning and evening meals. The dose can be increased to 10 mcg twice daily after 1 month of therapy. Each dose should be administered subcutaneously in the abdomen, thigh, or upper arm. When exenatide is added to metformin therapy, the current dose of metformin can be kept the same. When exenatide is added to sulfonylurea therapy, a reduction in the dose of sulfonylurea may be considered to reduce the risk of hypoglycemia.

Renal Impairment: Not recommended in patients with end-stage renal disease or severe renal impairment (creatinine clearance < 30 mL/min).

Hepatic Impairment: No dosage adjustment necessary.

Contraindications: Type 1 diabetes, end-stage renal disease or severe renal impairment (creatinine clearance < 30 mL/min), severe gastrointestinal disease.

Adverse Effects: Hypoglycemia, nausea, vomiting, diarrhea, feeling jittery, dizziness, headache, dyspepsia, acute pancreatitis.

Monitoring: HbA1c, FBG.

Drug Interactions: The effects of exenatide to slow gastric emptying may reduce the extent and rate of absorption of orally administered drugs, so it should be used with caution in patients receiving oral medications that require rapid gastrointestinal absorption. Medications that are dependent on threshold concentrations for efficacy, such as contraceptives, levothyroxine, and antibiotics, should be taken at least 1 hour before exenatide injection. If such drugs are to be administered with food, they should be taken with a meal or snack when exenatide is not administered.

Safety in Pregnancy: C

Comments: Exenatide is indicated for type 2 diabetic patients who are taking metformin, a sulfonylurea, or both, but have not achieved adequate glycemic control.

Dosage Forms: 5 and 10 mcg pre-filled pen injectors, 60 doses each

Website: www.byetta.com

Glimepiride (Amaryl)

Class: Sulfonylurea

Mechanism of Action: Sulfonylureas stimulate insulin release by blocking the energy-sensitive potassium channel of the beta cell. They also decrease hepatic glucose production and may improve insulin sensitivity at the receptor and post-receptor levels.

Clinical Effects: Sulfonylureas reduce HbA1c by up to 1-2% and fasting blood glucose by up to 60-80 mg/dL.

Dosage: Initial dose is 1-2 mg/day. May increase dose at 1-2 week intervals, with usual maintenance doses of 1-4 mg/day. Maximum dose is 8 mg/day. Elderly patients should be started at doses of 1 mg/day.

Renal Impairment: CrCl < 22 mL/min: initial dosage = 1 mg.

Hepatic Impairment: No data available.

Contraindications: Hypersensitivity, type 1 diabetes, diabetic ketoacidosis.

Adverse Effects: Headache, dizziness, weakness, nausea.

Monitoring: HbA1c, FBG.

Safety in Pregnancy: C

Dosage Forms: 1 mg, 2 mg, 4 mg tablets.

Website: www.amaryl.com

Glipizide (Glucotrol/Glucotrol XL)

Class: Sulfonylurea

Mechanism of Action: Sulfonylureas stimulate insulin release by blocking the energy-sensitive potassium channel of the beta cell. They also decrease hepatic glucose production and may improve insulin sensitivity at the receptor and post-receptor levels.

Clinical Effects: Sulfonylureas reduce HbA1c by up to 1-2% and fasting blood glucose by up to 60-80 mg/dL.

Dosage:

Glipizide (Glucotrol) is given at a starting dose of 5 mg, 30 minutes before a meal. Geriatric patients or those with liver disease may be started on 2.5 mg. Maintenance doses range from 2.5 to 40 mg/day; however doses above 20 mg generally do not provide greater blood glucose reduction and increase the risk of severe hypoglycemia. Single doses above 15 mg should be divided.

Glipizide-GITS (Glucotrol XL) Glipizide-GITS is given at a starting dose of 5 mg/day. Maintenance doses range from 5-20 mg/day.

Renal Impairment: No dosage adjustment necessary.

Hepatic Impairment: Initial dosage should be 2.5 mg/day.

Warnings/Contraindications: Sulfonylurea allergy, type 1 diabetes.

Adverse Effects: Headache, anorexia, nausea, vomiting, diarrhea, epigastric fullness, constipation, heartburn, rash, hives, photosensitivity, edema, hypoglycemia. Possible increased cardiovascular mortality.

Drug Interactions: Fluconazole increases levels of glipizide.

Monitoring: HbA1c, FBG.

Safety in Pregnancy: C

Comments: More effective when given 30 minutes before meals. When changing from immediate to sustained release, use same total daily dose.

Dosage Forms: 5 and 10 mg tablet; 5 and 10 mg extended-release tablets.

Website: www.pdr.net

Glipizide/Metformin (Metaglip)

Class: Sulfonylurea/biguanide

Mechanism of Action: Sulfonylureas stimulate insulin release by blocking the energy-sensitive potassium channel of the beta cell. They also decrease hepatic glucose production and may improve insulin sensitivity at the receptor and post-receptor levels. Metformin increases insulin sensitivity in the liver by inhibiting hepatic gluconeogenesis and/or glycogenolysis, thereby reducing hepatic glucose production. It also enhances muscle glucose uptake and utilization.

Clinical Effects: When used as initial therapy, Metaglip reduced HbA1c by up to 2.15% and fasting blood glucose by up to 55 mg/dL.

Dosage:

Initial therapy: 2.5/250 mg once a day with a meal; if FBG is 280-320 mg/dL, start with 2.5/500 mg twice a day with meals; may increase by one tablet per day every two weeks to a maximum of 10/2000 mg per day, given in divided doses.

Second-line therapy: (patients not controlled on a sulfonylurea or metformin alone): Start with 2.5/500 mg or 5/500 mg twice a day with meals; may increase up to a maximum of 20/2000 mg per day, given in divided doses.

Renal Impairment: Do not use in patients with renal insufficiency (serum creatinine $\geq$ 1.5 mg/dL in men or $\geq$ 1.4 mg/dL in women).

Hepatic Impairment: Do not use with severe liver disease.

Contraindications: Metformin should not be given to anyone ≥ 80 years of age without first documenting a normal creatinine clearance. Because of the metformin component, do not use in renal insufficiency (serum creatinine ≥ 1.5 mg/dL in men or ≥ 1.4 mg/dL in women), in patients receiving iodinated contrast material (discontinue temporarily for 48 hours after procedure because of potential for acute alteration of renal function, and do not resume until normal renal function has been documented), or in patients prone to metabolic acidosis or hypoxic states (liver failure, congestive heart failure requiring pharmacological therapy, diabetic ketoacidosis, major surgical procedures, sepsis, severe trauma, alcoholism, COPD); these conditions increase the risk of developing lactic acidosis. Not recommended for type 1 diabetes.

Adverse Effects: Anorexia, nausea, abdominal discomfort, diarrhea, metallic taste, vitamin B_{12} deficiency, lactic acidosis, hypoglycemia, headache, dizziness, rash, photosensitivity reactions. Possible increased cardiovascular mortality (sulfonylureas).

Drug Interactions: Fluconazole increases levels of glipizide; cimetidine increases blood levels of metformin

Monitoring: Renal function, HbA_{1c}, FBG, hematologic parameters (Hb, hematocrit, RBC indices).

Safety in Pregnancy: C

Comments: Give with meals. Patients already on glipizide and metformin may be switched to the nearest equivalent dose of the combination product.

Dosage Forms: 2.5/250 mg, 2.5/500 mg, 5/500 mg tablets.

Website: www.metaglip.com

Glyburide (DiaBeta, Micronase, Glynase)

Class: Sulfonylurea

Mechanism of Action: Sulfonylureas stimulate insulin release by blocking the energy-sensitive potassium channel of the beta cell. They also decrease hepatic glucose production and may improve insulin sensitivity at the receptor and post-receptor levels.

Clinical Effects: Sulfonylureas reduce HbA1c by up to 1-2% and fasting blood glucose by up to 60-80 mg/dL.

Dosage: Glyburide (DiaBeta/Micronase) is given at a starting dose of 2.5-5 mg daily; maintenance doses range from 2.5-20 mg/day in 1 or 2 divided doses. Glyburide (Glynase) has a starting dose of 1.5-3 mg daily; maintenance doses range from 3-12 mg/day in 1 or 2 divided doses.

Renal Impairment: CrCl 10-50 mL/min: use conservative initial and maintenance doses. CrCl < 10 mL/min: avoid use.

Hepatic Impairment: Use conservative initial and maintenance doses.

Contraindications: Hypersensitivity, type 1 diabetes.

Adverse Effects: Hypoglycemia, hypersensitivity, weight gain, nausea/abdominal pain. headache, dizziness, rash, photosensitivity reactions. Possible increased cardiovascular mortality.

Monitoring: HbA1c, FBG.

Safety in Pregnancy: C

Comments: Most effective when given 30 minutes before meals.

Dosage Forms: Diabeta: 1.25 mg, 2.5 mg, 5 mg tablets; Glynase: 1.5 mg, 3 mg micronized tablets.

Website: www.pdr.net

Glyburide/Metformin (Glucovance)

Class: Sulfonylurea/biguanide

Mechanism of Action: Sulfonylureas stimulate insulin release by blocking the energy-sensitive potassium channel of the beta cell. They also decrease hepatic glucose production and may improve insulin sensitivity at the receptor and post-receptor levels. Metformin increases insulin sensitivity in the liver by inhibiting hepatic gluconeogenesis and thereby reducing hepatic glucose production. It also enhances muscle glucose uptake and utilization.

Clinical Effects: When used as initial therapy in drug-naïve patients, Glucovance reduced HbA$_{1c}$ by up to 1.5% and fasting blood glucose by up to 50 mg/dL.

Dosage:

Initial therapy: 1.25/250 mg once or twice a day with meals. May titrate up to a total daily dose of 10/2000 mg. (Glucovance 5/500 mg should not be used as initial therapy due to risk of hypoglycemia.)

Second-line therapy (patients not adequately controlled on a sulfonylurea or metformin alone): 2.5/500 mg or 5/500 mg twice a day with meals. Maximum recommended daily dose is 20/2000 mg.

Renal Impairment: Do not use in patients with renal insufficiency (serum creatinine ≥ 1.5 mg/dL in men or ≥ 1.4 mg/dL in women).

Hepatic Impairment: Do not use with severe liver disease.

Contraindications: Metformin should not be given to anyone ≥ 80 years of age without first documenting a normal creatinine clearance. Because of the metformin component, do not use in renal insufficiency (serum creatinine ≥ 1.5 mg/dL in men or ≥ 1.4 mg/dL in women), in patients receiving iodinated contrast material (discontinue temporarily for 48 hours after procedure because of potential for acute alteration renal function, and do not resume until normal renal function has been documented), or in the presence of any condition associated with hypoxemia, dehydration, metabolic acidosis or sepsis (liver failure, binge drinking, congestive heart failure requiring pharmacological therapy, diabetic ketoacidosis, major surgical procedures, sepsis, severe trauma, alcoholism, binge drinking, COPD); these conditions increase the risk of developing lactic acidosis. Not recommended for type 1 diabetes.

Adverse Effects: Anorexia, nausea, abdominal discomfort, diarrhea, metallic taste, vitamin B_{12} deficiency, lactic acidosis, hypoglycemia, weight gain, headache, dizziness, rash, photosensitivity reactions. Possible increased cardiovascular mortality (sulfonylureas).

Monitoring: Renal function, HbA_{1c}, FBG, hematologic parameters (Hb, hematocrit, RBC indices).

Drug Interactions: Cimetidine increases blood levels of metformin.

Safety in Pregnancy: C

Comments: Give with meals. Patients already on glyburide and metformin may be switched to the nearest equivalent dose of the combination product.

Dosage Forms: 1.25/250 mg, 2.5/500 mg, 5/500 mg tablets.

Website: www.glucovance.com

Metformin (Glucophage/Glucophage XR, Glumetza, Fortamet)

Class: Biguanide

Mechanism of Action: Increases insulin sensitivity in the liver by inhibiting hepatic gluconeogenesis and/or glycogenolysis, thereby reducing hepatic glucose production. Metformin also enhances muscle glucose uptake and utilization.

Clinical Effects: Metformin reduces HbA1c by up to 1.5-2% and fasting blood glucose by up to 60-80 mg/dL.

Dosage: 500 mg tablet: starting dose is 500 mg twice a day with the morning and evening meals, up to a maximum of 2500 mg/day. 850 mg tablet: starting dose is 850 mg once daily with the largest meal, up to a maximum of 2550 mg/day. Dosage increases should be made in increments of one tablet every 2 weeks, up to a maximum of 2500 mg/day (2550 mg with 850 mg tablets).

Renal Impairment: Do not use in patients with renal insufficiency (serum creatinine $\geq$ 1.5 mg/dL in men or $\geq$ 1.4 mg/dL in women).

Hepatic Impairment: Do not use with severe liver disease.

Contraindications: Metformin should not be given to anyone $\geq$ 80 years of age without first documenting a normal creatinine clearance. Do not use in renal insufficiency (serum creatinine $\geq$ 1.5 mg/dL in men or $\geq$ 1.4 mg/dL in women), in patients receiving iodinated contrast material (discontinue temporarily for 48 hours after procedure because of potential for acute alteration of renal function, and do not resume until normal renal function has been documented), or in patients prone to metabolic acidosis or hypoxic states (liver failure, congestive heart failure requiring pharmacological therapy, diabetic ketoacidosis, major surgical procedures, sepsis, severe trauma, alcoholism, binge drinking, COPD); these conditions increase the risk of lactic acidosis.

Adverse Effects: Anorexia, nausea, abdominal discomfort, diarrhea, metallic taste, vitamin B_{12} deficiency, lactic acidosis.

Monitoring: Renal function, HbA1c, FBG, hematologic parameters (Hb, hematocrit, RBC indices).

Drug Interactions: Cimetidine increases blood levels of metformin.

Safety in Pregnancy: B
Comments: May be most useful in obese patients with dyslipidemia (decreases LDL and TG's); associated with no weight gain or mild weight loss. Approved for use down to 10 years of age.
Dosage Forms: Tablet: 500 mg, 850 mg, 1000 mg; Glucophage extended-release tablet: 500 mg, 750 mg; Glumetza extended-release tablet: 500 mg, 1000 mg
Website: www.pdr.net

Miglitol (Glyset)

Class: Alpha-glucosidase inhibitor
Mechanism of Action: These drugs act locally in the small intestine by inhibiting alpha-glucosidase enzymes; this action slows digestion of ingested carbohydrates, delays glucose absorption, and reduces the increase in postprandial blood glucose.
Dosage: 25 mg three times/day with the first bite of each main meal. Maintenance dose ranges are 50-100 mg three times/day. Dose adjustments should be made at 4-8 week intervals.
Clinical Effects: Alpha-glucosidase inhibitors cause a 0.5-1% reduction in HbA1c and have no significant effect on fasting blood glucose levels.
Renal Impairment: Primarily excreted by the kidneys; little information in patients with a CrCl < 25 mL/min.
Hepatic Impairment: No dosage adjustment is necessary.
Contraindications: Major GI disorders, including inflammatory bowel disease,

chronic ulceration, malabsorption, or partial intestinal obstruction.
Adverse Effects: Abdominal bloating, flatulence, diarrhea, rash. Adverse GI effects tend to diminish with continued treatment.
Monitoring: HbA1c, FBG.
Drug Interactions: Decreases absorption and bioavailability of digoxin and propranolol; digestive enzymes (amylase, pancreatin), intestinal adsorbents (charcoal) reduce effects of miglitol.
Safety in Pregnancy: B
Comments: Most effective in patients with postprandial hyperglycemia; not associated with weight gain or hypoglycemia; must use glucose and not complex sugars to reverse hypoglycemia, if it occurs
Dosage Forms: 25 mg, 50 mg, 100 mg tablets.
Website: www.glyset.com

Nateglinide (Starlix)

Class: Meglitinide (phenylalanine derivative)
Mechanism of Action: Meglitinides stimulate insulin release from pancreatic beta cells in response to a glucose load (meal). Insulin release is glucose dependent and diminishes at low glucose concentrations. There are distinct beta cell binding sites for nateglinide apart from the sulfonylurea binding site.
Clinical Effects: Nateglinide lowers HbA1c by up to 1% but has no significant effect on fasting blood glucose.

Dosage: Nateglinide has an initial and maintenance dose of 120 mg three times/day. If a patient is close to HbA1c goal, the dose may be started at 60 mg three times/day. Doses should be given 1-30 minutes before meals. The number of doses is based on the number of meals eaten. If a meal is skipped, that dose should be omitted. At least 1 week should elapse between dosage adjustments.

Renal Impairment: No dosage adjustment necessary.

Hepatic Impairment: Use with caution in patients with severe liver disease.

Contraindications: Hypersensitivity, type 1 diabetes, diabetic ketoacidosis with or without coma.

Adverse Effects: Hypoglycemia, headache, nausea, diarrhea, constipation, dizziness.

Monitoring: HbA1c, FBG.

Drug Interactions: No significant interactions.

Safety in Pregnancy: C

Comments: Most effective for lowering postprandial blood glucose.

Dosage Forms: 60 mg, 120 mg tablets.

Website: www.starlix.com

Pioglitazone (Actos)

Class: Thiazolidinedione

Mechanism of Action: Pioglitazone decreases insulin resistance in muscle and adipose tissue by activating the peroxisome proliferator-activated receptor gamma, which increases transcription of proteins involved in glucose uptake. It also decreases hepatic glucose production by improving hepatic insulin sensitivity, and preserves pancreatic beta-cell function.

Clinical Effects: Thiazolidinediones reduce HbA1c by up to 0.6-1.9 % and fasting blood glucose by up to 50-80 mg/dL.

Dosage: Pioglitazone has a starting dose of 15 mg/day with maintenance doses of 15-45 mg/day given as a single dose. May be given without regard to meals.

Renal Impairment: No dosage adjustment necessary.

Hepatic Impairment: Do not use in patients with active liver disease or increased serum transaminase levels (ALT > 2.5 x upper limit of normal).

Adverse Effects: Weight gain, edema, headache, myalgia, upper respiratory tract infection, anemia, macular edema (rare), increased frequency of upper limb fractures.

Warnings/Contraindications: Class III or IV heart failure (not recommended due to fluid retention), liver disease, type 1 diabetes (ineffective without insulin).

Drug Interactions: Effects of oral contraceptives and statins may be decreased based on data from another thiazolidinedione; additional caution regarding contraception is needed. Pioglitazone may be a weak inducer of CYP3A4.

Monitoring: HbA1c, FBG.

Safety in Pregnancy: C

Comments: May result in ovulation in premenopausal anovulatory women. It may take several weeks for onset of action and several months for peak activity. Requires the presence of insulin for action.

Dosage Forms: 15 mg, 30 mg, 45 mg

tablets.
Website: www.actos.com

Pioglitazone/Glimepiride (Duetact)

Class: Thiazolidinedione/sulfonylurea
Mechanism of Action: Pioglitazone decreases insulin resistance in muscle and adipose tissue by activating the peroxisome proliferator-activated receptor gamma, which increases transcription of proteins involved in glucose uptake. It also decreases hepatic glucose production by improving hepatic insulin sensitivity. Sulfonylureas stimulate insulin secretion by blocking the energy-sensitive potassium channel of the beta cell. They also decrease hepatic glucose production and may improve insulin sensitivity at the receptor and post-receptor levels.
Clinical Effects: When pioglitazone is added to a sulfonylurea, the fasting blood glucose is decreased by up to 40-60 mg/dL and the HbA1c is reduced by up to 0.9-1.7%.
Dosage: Initial dose is 30/2 mg once daily in patients previously on monotherapy with a sulfonylurea or pioglitazone. May increase dose at 1-2 week intervals, but in patients previously treated with sulfonylurea monotherapy, it may take 2-3 months to see the full effect of the pioglitazone component. Maximum recommended daily dose is 45 mg of pioglitazone and 8 mg of glimepiride.
Renal Impairment: Initial dosing should be conservative.

Hepatic Impairment: Do not use in patients with active liver disease or increased serum transaminase levels (ALT > 2.5 x upper limit of normal).
Warnings and Contraindications: Class III or IV heart failure (not recommended due to fluid retention), liver disease, type 1 diabetes mellitus (ineffective without insulin), diabetic ketoacidosis.
Adverse Effects: Weight gain, edema, fluid retention, hypoglycemia, headache, dizziness, weakness, nausea, myalgia, macular edema (rare), anemia, increased frequency of upper limb fractures, osteoporosis.
Drug Interactions: Effects of oral contraceptives and statins may be decreased; additional caution regarding contraception is needed. Pioglitazone may be a weak inducer of CYP3A4.
Monitoring: HbA1c, FBG.
Safety in Pregnancy: C
Comments: May result in ovulation in premenopausal anovulatory women. It may take several weeks for onset of action and several months for peak activity of pioglitazone component. Should be given once daily with the first meal of the day.
Dosage Forms: 30/2 mg, 30/4 mg tablets
Website: www.duetact.com

Pioglitazone/Metformin (ACTOplus met)

Class: Thiazolidinedione/biguanide
Mechanism of Action: Pioglitazone decreases insulin resistance in muscle and adipose tissue by activating the peroxisome proliferator-activated receptor gamma, which increases

transcription of proteins involved in glucose uptake. It also decreases hepatic glucose production by improving hepatic insulin sensitivity. Metformin increases insulin sensitivity in the liver by inhibiting hepatic gluconeogenesis and/or glycogenolysis, thereby reducing hepatic glucose production. It also enhances muscle glucose uptake and utilization.

Clinical Effects: When pioglitazone is added to metformin, the fasting blood glucose is decreased by up to 40-50 mg/dL and the HbA1c is reduced by up to 1%.

Dosage: Initial dose is 15/500 mg or 15/850 mg once or twice daily with meals in patients on metformin monotherapy. For patients on pioglitazone mono-therapy, the initial dose should be 15/500 mg twice daily or 15/850 mg once daily. Patients switching from combination therapy with pioglitazone plus metformin as separate tablets may be started on either the 15/500 mg or 15/850 mg tablet strengths based on the doses of each medication already being taken. Doses should be given with meals and titrated gradually. Maximum recommended daily dose is 45 mg of pioglitazone and 2550 mg of metformin.

Renal Impairment: Do not use in patients with renal insufficiency (serum creatinine ≥ 1.5 mg/dL in men or ≥ 1.4 mg/dL in women).

Hepatic Impairment: Do not use in patients with active liver disease or increased serum transaminase levels (ALT > 2.5 x upper limit of normal).

Contraindications: Metformin should not be given to anyone ≥ 80 years of age without first documenting a normal creatinine clearance. Because of the metformin component, do not use in renal insufficiency (serum creatinine ≥ 1.5 mg/dL in men or ≥ 1.4 mg/dL in women); in patients receiving iodinated contrast material (discontinue temporarily for 48 hours after procedure because of potential for acute alteration of renal function, and do not resume until normal renal function has been documented); or in patients prone to metabolic acidosis or hypoxic states (liver failure, congestive heart failure requiring pharmacological therapy, diabetic ketoacidosis, major surgical procedures, sepsis, severe trauma, alcoholism, binge drinking, COPD); these conditions increase the risk of developing lactic acidosis. Not recommended for type 1 diabetes, Class III or IV heart failure (due to fluid retention).

Adverse Effects: Weight gain, edema, fluid retention, myalgia, nausea, anorexia, abdominal discomfort, diarrhea, metallic taste, vitamin B12 deficiency, lactic acidosis, macular edema (rare), increased frequency of upper limb fractures.

Drug Interactions: Effects of oral contraceptives and statins may be decreased by pioglitazone; additional caution regarding contraception is needed. Pioglitazone may also be a weak inducer of CYP3A4. Cimetidine increases blood levels of metformin.

Monitoring: HbA1c, FBG, renal function, hematologic parameters (Hb, hematocrit, RBC indices).

Safety in Pregnancy: C

Comments: May result in ovulation in premenopausal anovulatory women. It may take several weeks for onset of action and several months for peak activity of pioglitazone component.

Dosage Forms: 15/500 mg, 15/850 mg tablets

Website: www.actoplusmet.com

Pramlintide (Symlin)

Class: Amylin mimetic

Mechanism of Action: Amylin is a neuroendocrine hormone secreted with insulin by pancreatic beta cells in response to food intake and subsequent elevations in blood glucose. Pramlintide is an amylin mimetic that slows gastric emptying, reducing the rate at which glucose appears in the bloodstream; decreases postprandial hepatic glucose output by suppressing glucagon secretion; and decreases food intake by enhancing satiety, potentially leading to weight loss.

Clinical Effects: Type 1 diabetes: Lowers HbA1c by 0.18-0.33%, reduces weight by 1.1-3.0 kg, and reduces total, short-acting, and long-acting insulin by up to 12%, 21.7%, and 0.4%, respectively. Type 2 diabetes: Lowers HbA1c by 0.4-0.56%, reduces weight by 1.5-2.76 kg, reduces total, short-acting, and long-acting insulin by up to 6.4%, 10.3%, and 4.2%, respectively.

Dosage: Type 1 diabetes: Starting dose is 15 mcg subcutaneously before each major meal (at least 250 calories or 30 gm carbohydrates). Reduce pre-meal insulin dose (rapid-acting, short-acting, and fixed-mix [70/30] insulin) by 50%. Increase pramlintide in 15 mcg increments to a maintenance dose of 30-60 mcg before major meals. Dose increases should be made when there is no nausea for 3 days. If nausea persists at the 45 or 60 mcg doses, reduce dose to 30 mcg. If the 30 mcg dose is not tolerated, consider discontinuing. Adjust insulin dose once patient is on a stable pramlintide regimen.

Type 2 diabetes: Starting dose is 60 mcg subcutaneously before each major meal (at least 250 calories or 30 gm carbohydrates). Reduce pre-meal insulin dose (rapid-acting, short-acting, and fixed-mix [70/30] insulin) by 50%. Increase pramlintide to 120 mcg when there is no nausea for 3-7 days. If nausea persists at the 120 mcg dose, reduce dose to 60 mcg. Adjust insulin dose once patient is on a stable pramlintide regimen.

Administration: Pramlintide and insulin should always be administered as separate injections. It should not be mixed with any type of insulin and should be given subcutaneously into the abdomen or thigh.

Renal Impairment: No dosage adjustment is necessary if creatinine clearance >20 mL/min. Has not been studied in patients on hemodialysis.

Hepatic Impairment: Not studied in patients with hepatic insufficiency. Hepatic dysfunction is not expected to affect blood concentrations since pramlintide undergoes mostly renal metabolism.

Monitoring: HbA1c, FBG.

Warnings/Contraindications: Pramlintide is used with insulin and has been associated with an increased risk of insulin-induced hypoglycemia, particularly in patients with Type 1 diabetes. When severe hypoglycemia with pramlintide occurs, it is seen within 3 hours following a pramlintide injection. Appropriate patient selection, careful patient instruction, and insulin dose adjustments are critical elements for reducing this risk. Contraindications include hypersensitivity to pramlintide or any of its components, including metacresol; gastroparesis; hypoglycemia unawareness.

Adverse Effects: Hypoglycemia, nausea, headache, anorexia, vomiting, abdominal pain, fatigue

Drug Interactions: Due to its effects on gastric emptying, pramlintide should not be used with drugs that alter gastrointestinal motility or slow intestinal absorption. It may delay the absorption of oral medications taken concurrently, so if a drug requires a rapid onset or is dependent on threshold concentrations for efficacy, such as levothyroxine, it should be taken 1 hour prior to or 2 hours after pramlintide is given.

Safety in Pregnancy: C

Comments: Pramlintide is indicated as an adjunct treatment for type 1 diabetes patients who use mealtime insulin and have failed to achieve adequate glycemic control. It is also indicated for type 2 diabetes patients who use mealtime insulin and have failed to achieve adequate glycemic control, with or without a concurrent sulfonylurea and/or metformin.

Dosage Forms: 5 ml vial (60 mcg/mL). Unopened vials should be kept refrigerated prior to use. The vial may be kept at room temperature or refrigerated once opened and should be used within 28 days.

Website: www.symlin.com

Repaglinide (Prandin)

Class: Meglitinide (benzoic acid derivative)

Mechanism of Action: Meglitinides stimulate insulin release from pancreatic beta cells in response to a glucose load (meal). Insulin release is glucose dependent and diminishes at low glucose concentrations. There are distinct beta cell binding sites for repaglinide apart from the sulfonylurea binding site.

Clinical Effects: Repaglinide lowers HbA1c by up to 1-2% and fasting blood glucose by up to 60-80 mg/dL.

Dosage: For patients not previously treated or whose HbA1c < 8%, the starting dose should be 0.5 mg with each meal; if patient has previously been treated with blood-glucose lowering agents or whose HbA1c > 8%, the initial dose is 1 or 2 mg with each meal. The dosage range is 0.5-4 mg with each meal (maximum daily dose = 16 mg). The number of doses is based on the number of meals eaten, and should be given within 15 minutes of each meal. If a meal is skipped, that dose should be omitted. At least 1 week should elapse between dosage adjustments.

Renal Impairment: CrCl = 20-40 mL/min: initiate with 0.5 mg with meals and titrate carefully.

Hepatic Impairment: Use conservative initial and maintenance doses; use longer intervals between dose adjustments.

Contraindications: Hypersensitivity, type 1 diabetes, diabetic ketoacidosis with or without coma.

Adverse Effects: Hypoglycemia, headache, nausea/vomiting/diarrhea, constipation, dyspepsia.

Monitoring: HbA1c, FBG.

Drug Interactions: CYP2C9 and CYP3A3/4 enzyme substrate. Agents that inhibit or induce these enzymes may increase repaglinide concentrations. Gemfibrozil and itraconazole increase levels of repaglinide (not recommended for concurrent use).

Safety in Pregnancy: C

Comments: Most effective for decreasing postprandial blood glucose

Dosage Forms: 0.5 mg, 1 mg, 2 mg tablets.

Website: www.prandin.com

Rosiglitazone (Avandia)

Class: Thiazolidinedione

Mechanism of Action: Rosiglitazone decreases insulin resistance in muscle and adipose tissue by activating the peroxisome proliferator-activated receptor gamma, which increases transcription of proteins involved in glucose uptake. It also decreases hepatic glucose production by improving hepatic insulin sensitivity, and preserves pancreatic beta-cell function.

Clinical Effects: Thiazolidinediones reduce HbA1c by up to 0.6-1.9 % and fasting blood glucose by up to 50-80 mg/dL.

Dosage: Rosiglitazone has a starting dose of 4 mg/day, with maintenance doses of 2-8 mg/day given in 1 or 2 divided doses. Dosage increases may be made if patients have inadequate response following 8-12 weeks of treatment.

Renal Impairment: No dose adjustment necessary.

Hepatic Impairment: Do not use if patient has active live disease or increased serum transaminase levels (ALT > 2.5 x upper limit of normal).

Monitoring: HbA1c, FBG.

Drug Interactions: Gemfibrozil and other inhibitors of CYP2C8 may increase rosiglitazone concentrations; rifampin and other inducers of CYP2C8 may decrease rosiglitazone concentrations.

Warnings/Contraindications: Symptomatic heart failure (not recommended), NYHA Class III or IV heart failure (contraindicated); after initiation or dose increase of rosiglitazone, observe patients for heart failure (if CHF develops, treat accordingly and consider dose reduction or discontinuation of rosiglitazone) Do not initiate if active liver disease or increased serum transaminases. Not recommended for type 1 diabetes (ineffective without insulin). Not recommended for patients already receiving insulin therapy or nitrates. A meta-analysis of 42 clinical studies (mean duration 6 months; 14,237 total patients), most of which compared rosiglitazone to placebo, showed rosiglitazone to be associated with an increased risk of myocardial ischemic events such as angina or myocardial infarction. Three other studies (mean duration 41 months; 14,067 total patients), comparing rosiglitazone to some other approved oral antidiabetic agents or placebo, have not confirmed or excluded this risk. In two, recent, randomized intensive vs. standard glycemic control trials (ADVANCE, VADT), rosiglitazone was not associated with increased MI or cardiovascular mortality. In their entirety, the available data on the risk of myocardial ischemia are inconclusive.

Adverse Effects: Weight gain, fluid retention, headache, anemia, macular edema (rare), increased frequency of bone fracture in female patients, acute lowering of HDL in combination with fibrates.

Safety in Pregnancy: C

Comments: It may take several weeks for onset of action and several months for peak activity. Requires the presence of insulin for action. Approved for use in triple combination therapy (with secretagogue plus metformin).

Dosage Forms: 2 mg, 4 mg, 8 mg tablets.

Website: www.avandia.com

Rosiglitazone/Glimepiride (Avandaryl)

Class: Thiazolidinedione/sulfonylurea

Mechanism of Action: Rosiglitazone decreases insulin resistance in muscle and adipose tissue by activating the peroxisome proliferator-activated receptor gamma, which increases transcription of proteins involved in glucose uptake. It also decreases hepatic glucose production by improving hepatic insulin sensitivity. Sulfonylureas stimulate insulin secretion by blocking the energy-sensitive potassium channel of the beta cell. They also decrease hepatic glucose production and may improve insulin sensitivity at the receptor and post-receptor levels.

Clinical Effects: When rosiglitazone is added to a sulfonylurea, the fasting blood glucose is decreased by up to 40-65 mg/dL and the HbA1c is reduced by up to 0.9-1.5%.

Dosage: Initial dose is 4/1 mg or 4/2 mg once daily in patients previously on monotherapy with a sulfonylurea or rosiglitazone. For patients previously treated with rosiglitazone monotherapy, the dose of Avandaryl may be increased by increasing the glimepiride component in no more than 2 mg increments at 1-2 week intervals. For patients previously treated with sulfonylurea monotherapy, it may take 2 weeks to see a reduction in blood glucose and 2-3 months to see the full effect of the rosiglitazone component. If additional glucose control is needed, the dose of the glimepiride component may be increased. Maximum recommended daily dose is 8 mg of rosiglitazone and 4 mg of glimepiride.

Renal Impairment: Initial dosing should be conservative.

Hepatic Impairment: Do not use in patients with active liver disease or increased serum transaminases (ALT > 2.5 x upper limit of normal).

Warnings and Contraindications: See warnings/contraindications for rosiglitazone, p. 182.

Adverse Effects: Weight gain, fluid retention, hypoglycemia, headache, dizziness, weakness, nausea, macular edema (rare), increased frequency of bone fracture in female patients, acute lowering of HDL in combination with fibrates.

Drug Interactions: Gemfibrozil increases rosiglitazone concentrations; rifampin decreases rosiglitazone concentrations.

Monitoring: HbA1c, FBG.

Safety in Pregnancy: C

Comments: May result in ovulation in premenopausal anovulatory women. It may take several weeks for onset of action and several months for peak activity of rosiglitazone component.

Dosage Forms: 4/1 mg, 4/2 mg, 4/4 mg tablets

Website: www.avandaryl.com

Rosiglitazone/Metformin (Avandamet)

Class: Thiazolidinedione/biguanide

Mechanism of Action: Rosiglitazone decreases insulin resistance in muscle and adipose tissue by activating the peroxisome proliferator-activated receptor-gamma, which increases transcription of proteins involved in glucose uptake. It also decreases hepatic glucose production by improving hepatic insulin sensitivity, and preserves pancreatic beta-cell function. Metformin increases insulin sensitivity in the liver by inhibiting hepatic gluconeogenesis and/or glycogenolysis, thereby reducing hepatic glucose production. It also enhances muscle glucose uptake and utilization.

Dosage: If patient's metformin dose was 1000 mg/day, start with 2/500 mg twice a day with meals. If patient's metformin dose was 2000 mg/day, start with 2/1000 mg twice a day with meals. If patient's rosiglitazone dose was 4 mg/day, start with 2/500 mg twice a day with meals. If patient's rosiglitazone dose was 8 mg/day, start with 4/500 mg twice a day with meals. If patients have inadequate response, metformin dosage increases may be made after 1-2 weeks and rosiglitazone dosage increases may be made after 8-12 weeks of treatment. Maximum recommended daily dose is 8/2000 mg.

Renal Impairment: Metformin should not be given to anyone over the age of 80 without first documenting a normal creatinine clearance. Because of the metformin component, do not use in patients with renal insufficiency (serum creatinine $\geq$ 1.5 mg/dL in men or $\geq$ 1.4 mg/dL in women).

Hepatic Impairment: Do not use if patient has active live disease or increased serum transaminase levels (ALT > 2.5x upper limit of normal).

Monitoring: HbA$_{1c}$, FBG, renal function, hematologic parameters.

Drug Interactions: Gemfibrozil increases rosiglitazone concentrations; rifampin decreases rosiglitazone concentrations. Cimetidine increases metformin concentrations.

Warnings and Contraindications: See warnings/contraindications for rosiglitazone, p. 182. Acute or chronic metabolic acidosis, renal insufficiency (serum creatinine ≥ 1.5 mg/dL in men or ≥ 1.4 mg/dL in women), patients receiving iodinated contrast material (discontinue temporarily for 48 hours after procedure because of potential for acute alteration of renal function, and do not resume until normal renal function has been documented), patients prone to metabolic acidosis or hypoxic states (liver failure, congestive heart failure requiring pharmacological therapy, diabetic ketoacidosis, major surgical procedures, sepsis, severe trauma, alcoholism, binge drinking, COPD); these conditions increase the risk of lactic acidosis.

Adverse Effects: Weight gain, fluid retention, hepatotoxicity, anemia, headache, anorexia, nausea, abdominal discomfort, diarrhea, metallic taste, vitamin B_{12} deficiency, lactic acidosis, macular edema, increased frequency of bone fracture in female patients, acute lowering of HDL in combination with fibrates.

Safety in Pregnancy: C

Comments: May result in ovulation in premenopausal anovulatory women. It may take several weeks for onset of action and several months for peak activity. Requires the presence of insulin for action.

Dosage Forms: 1/500 mg, 2/500 mg, 4/500 mg, 2/1000 mg, 4/1000 mg tablets.

Website: www.avandamet.com

Sitagliptin (Januvia)

Class: Dipeptidyl peptidase-4 (DPP-4) inhibitor

Mechanism of Action: Glucagon-like peptide-1 (GLP-1) and glucose-dependent insulinotropic polypeptide (GIP) are incretin hormones that are released from cells in the intestine in response to food. They bind to receptors on pancreatic beta cells, stimulating the release of insulin and reducing the release of glucagon. Sitagliptin works by inhibiting DPP-4, an enzyme that rapidly breaks down GLP-1 and GIP. The incretin system is impaired in type 2 diabetics, so sitagliptin enhances its function, leading to decreased blood sugar levels as well as preserving beta-cell function.

Clinical Efficacy: Sitagliptin reduces HbA_{1c} by 0.7-1.5% when used as monotherapy and by up to 2.9% when used in combination with metformin or a thiazolidinedione. It also decreases fasting blood glucose by up to 25 mg/dL.

Dosage: 100 mg once daily as monotherapy or in combination with metformin or a thiazolidinedione.

Renal Impairment: CrCl 30-50 mL/min: 50 mg/day; CrCl < 30 mL/min or ESRD (on dialysis): 25 mg/day.

Hepatic Impairment: No dosage adjustment necessary.

Adverse Effects: Nasopharyngitis, headache, upper respiratory tract infection, skin allergic reactions including Stevens-Johnson Syndrome (erythema multiforme).

Monitoring: HbA$_{1c}$, FBG, renal function.

Drug Interactions: Slight increase in digoxin concentrations in patients on 100 mg dose of sitagliptin.

Safety in Pregnancy: B

Comments: Not associated with weight gain.

Dosage Forms: 25 mg, 50 mg, 100 mg tablets.

Website: www.januvia.com

Sitagliptin/Metformin (Janumet)

Class: Dipeptidyl peptidase-4 (DPP-4) inhibitor/biguanide

Mechanism of Action: See sitagliptin (p. 185) and metformin (p. 175).

Clinical Efficacy: When sitagliptin is added to metformin, the HbA$_{1c}$ is reduced by an additional 0.6%-0.8% compared to sitagliptin alone. The fasting blood glucose is also reduced by an additional 20-35 mg/dL.

Dosage: Initial dose is 50/500 mg twice a day with meals; may increase to 50/1000 mg twice a day. For patients on metformin alone, the recommended starting dose should equal sitagliptin 50 mg twice a day and the dose of metformin already being taken. Patients taking metformin 850 mg twice a day should be started on Janumet 50/1000 mg twice a day. For patients already on sitagliptin and metformin, Janumet may be initiated at the dose of sitagliptin and metformin already being taken.

Renal Impairment: Do not use in renal insufficiency (serum creatinine ≥ 1.5 mg/dL in men or ≥ 1.4 mg/dl in women) due to metformin component.

Hepatic Impairment: Do not use with severe liver disease.

Contraindications: Metformin should not be given to anyone ≥ 80 years of age without first documenting a normal creatinine clearance. Because of the metformin component, do not use in renal insufficiency (serum creatinine ≥ 1.5 mg/dL in men or ≥ 1.4 mg/dL in women); in patients receiving iodinated contrast material (discontinue temporarily for 48 hours after procedure because of potential for acute alteration of renal function, and do not resume until normal renal function has been documented); or in patients prone to metabolic acidosis or hypoxic states (liver failure, congestive heart failure requiring pharmacological therapy, diabetic ketoacidosis, major surgical procedures, sepsis, severe trauma, alcoholism, binge drinking, COPD); these conditions increase the risk of developing lactic acidosis.

Adverse Effects: Headache, upper respiratory tract infection, nausea, vomiting, abdominal pain, lactic acidosis.

Monitoring: HbA$_{1c}$, FBG, renal function, LFTs (baseline and periodically thereafter), hematologic parameters (Hb, hematocrit, RBC indices)

Drug Interactions: Digoxin: slight increase in digoxin concentrations in patients on 100 mg dose of sitagliptin. Cimetidine increases blood levels of metformin.

Safety in Pregnancy: B

Comments: Not associated with weight gain. Give with meals.
Dosage Forms: 50/500 mg, 50/1000 mg tablets
Website: www.janumet.com

Insulin*

Mechanism of Action: Main hormone required for proper glucose utilization and metabolic processes. Categorized by onset, duration, and intensity of action
Adverse Effects: Hypoglycemia, local reactions (itching, edema, stinging, pain or warmth at injection site, atrophy or hypertrophy of subcutaneous fat tissue).
Safety in Pregnancy: B, except for glargine (Lantus), detemir (Levemir), aspart (Novolog) and glulisine (Apidra), which are category C.
Compatibility of Insulin Preparations, Timing of Administration, Dosage Forms (Injections): See Tables 11.2 and 11.3, pp. 187-188.
Website: www.pdr.net

Table 11.2. Insulin Products

Insulin	Onset	Peak	Duration
Rapid-acting			
Lispro (Humulog)	5-15 min	30-90 min	5 h
Aspart (Novolog)	5-15 min	30-90 min	5 h
Glulisine (Apidra)	5-15 min	30-90 min	5 h
Inhaled (Exubera) (no longer available in US)	10-20 min	30-90 min	5-8 h
Short-acting			
Regular U100 (Humulin R/Novolin R)	30-60 min	2-3 h	5-8 h
Regular U500 (concentrated)	30-60 min	2-3 h	5-8 h
Intermediate-acting			
Isophane insulin (NPH = Humulin N/Novolin N)	2-4 h	4-10 h	10-16 h
Long-acting			
Glargine (Lantus)	2-4 h	6-8 h	10-24 h
Detemir (Levemir)	2-4 h	6-8 h	6-23 h
Premixed			
70% NPH/30% regular (Humulin 70/30, Novolin 70/30)	30-60 min	dual	10-16 h
50% NPH/50% regular (Humulin 50/50)	30-60 min	dual	10-16 h
75% NPL/25% lispro (Humulog Mix 75/25)	5-15 min	dual	10-16 h
50% NPL/50% lispro (Humulog Mix 50/50)	5-15 min	dual	10-16 h
70% NPA/30% aspart (Novolog Mix)	5-15 min	dual	10-16 h

NPH = neutral protamine Hagedorn, NPL = insulin lispro protamine, NPA = insulin aspart protamine. Adapted from: JAMA 2003;289:2254-2264.

Table 11.3. Compatibility and Timing of Insulin Products

Compatibility of Insulin Preparations
Lispro (Humulog): Compatible with NPH
Aspart (Novolog): Compatible with NPH
Regular insulin: Compatible with NPH if given ≤ 5 minutes after mixing
Isophane insulin suspension (NPH): Compatible with regular insulin, lispro, aspart
Glargine (Lantus): Should not be mixed with other insulins

Timing of Administration
Rapid-acting (lispro, aspart, glulisine, inhaled): Given 1-15 min before a meal (usually 5 min)
Short-acting (regular): Given 30-60 min before a meal
Intermediate-acting (NPH): Given 2 times per day
Long-acting (glargine, detemir): Given once a day

Index